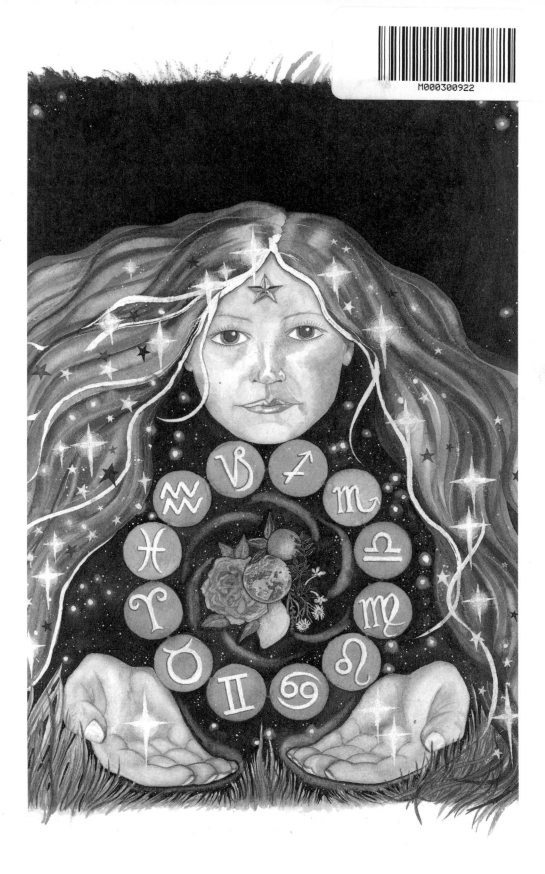

First published in Great Britain in 2002
by The C.W. Daniel Company Limited
1 Church Path, Saffron Walden,
Essex, CB10 1JP, United Kingdom

© Patricia Davis 2002
Illustrations © Diane Melanie 2002

ISBN 0 85207 356 9

Other Books by Patricia Davis:

Aromatherapy: An A-Z

A Change for the Better

Subtle Aromatherapy

Produced in association with
Book Production Consultants plc, 25-27 High Street,
Chesterton, Cambridge, CB4 1ND.
Designed by Marion Hughston.
Printing by The Cromwell Press, Trowbridge, Wiltshire.

Patricia Davis
Astrological Aromatherapy

Illustrated By Diane Melanie
Index Compiled by Ann Griffiths

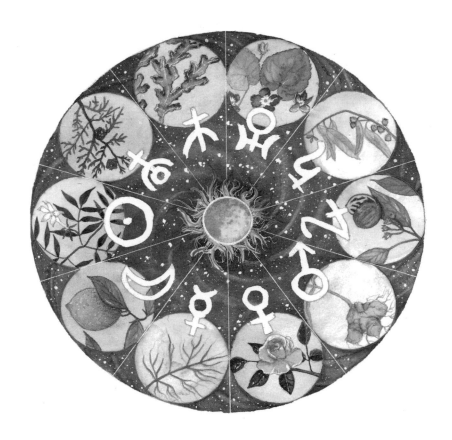

SAFFRON WALDEN
THE C.W. DANIEL COMPANY LIMITED

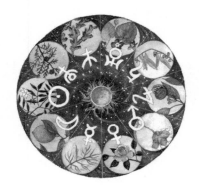

This book is dedicated to Evelyn Burges,
friend, astrologer and tarot reader extraordinaire.

Astrological Aromatherapy

Acknowledgements

My thanks, first of all, to all the teachers who have shaped my understanding of astrology: Ron Gwynn and tutors of the Faculty of Astrological Studies who taught me the basics; and Evelyn Burges, Derek Hawkins, David Matthews and others who have helped me refine them over the past decade; also to Maia MacTiernan for permission to reproduce her table of Chiron transits and to David Matthews for technical advice.

I am grateful to all the therapists and others who completed questionnaires to help with my research, especially to Totnes Natural Health Centre and to Teresa Knight, also to the many volunteers who tried out the Zodiac blends.

My profound thanks to Diane Melanie for the intuition and sensitivity she brought to making the inspired illustrations and the excitement and fun we had collaborating on this project.

Finally, an enormous thank you to Evelyn Burges for reading the manuscript with truly Virgoan thoroughness and making many thoughtful suggestions, lending me books and ferreting out obscure but relevant volumes in bookshops, but most of all for her enthusiasm, support and encouragement throughout the writing process.

Totnes, Devon,
November 2001

Astrological Aromatherapy

Contents

How it all began

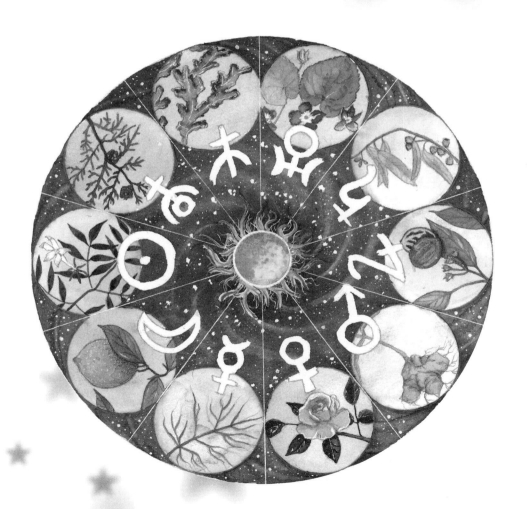

How it all began

"Anything that is born in a moment of time takes on the qualities of that moment of time."

CARL JUNG.

How *did* it all begin? How do aromatherapy and astrology connect with each other?

Rather than try to answer those questions straight away, I invite you to come with me on a journey back through time. How much time, we do not know, but it is certainly many, many thousands of years. So find somewhere comfortable to sit or lie, close your eyes and come with me to a time when the world was young:

Imagine that you are sitting on a hillside, under a brilliant starry sky. You are young, just on the verge of puberty. Behind you is a comfortable rock that you can lean against, beside you is an elder of your clan, perhaps your grandmother or grandfather. This is the very first time that you have been chosen to be part of the night guard and you feel maybe a little nervous but very proud and excited. Down below you can see the hide-covered shelters where your people are sleeping and the faint glow of the fire which has been built up for the night, as much to keep any marauding animals away as to allow the women a quick start to making hot food in the morning, for the winter is not quite over and some grains or berries heated over the embers are still welcome before a day spent foraging or hunting.

The Moon is large and low on the horizon and after a while the wise old one beside you asks, "How many days do you think, young 'un, before the Moon will be full?" You stare at the silver light for a minute or two before answering, "About three days, I think." "Well done, young 'un, I think four days, but that was a good guess. Now, when she is full it will be time to check all the spears and have five or six people on watch all day as well as all night because it will be the fourth Full Moon since the dark time when the night was longest and that means that the bison herds will be coming through the valley very soon."

You nod. You don't need to be told how important it is to kill as many bison as possible during the migrations. You're wearing bison leather on your feet, you sleep under a roof of their hide at night, and bison meat roasted over the fire is the best food you have ever tasted. Idly, you pick a blade of grass and twist it round your fingers, noticing its pungent scent. Your wise old companion notices it, too, and says, "Hey! Don't waste that grass, it's a good medicine. We'll pick some to take down to your mother for drying in the morning, but not too much because it will grow a great deal more by the time of the next Moon and it will be better to pick a good lot then. You can usually find it growing around here when those stars are above the top of the biggest hill...Do you see them? The ones that look like a bull?" And you follow the pointing finger and make out the shape of the animal in the sky.

Of course, that is conjecture, but there is plenty of evidence to suggest that it is very close to the truth. Animal bones with the Moon's phases scratched into them have been found at ancient living sites and dated to around 37,000 years old. In some very early burials, medicinal herbs have been found alongside human remains and identified from their fossilised pollens: there were as many as 22 plants that we know to be of medicinal value in one grave, which may have been that of a medicine man. The way of life of the few peoples who still live in close harmony with nature gives us many insights into the lives of our distant ancestors, too. There are not many of them left now, but fortunately we have some anthropological studies made in the earlier part of the last century.

Certainly the Moon was a major aid to keeping track of time. The Sun was our first clock, dividing time into day and night and marking the passage of the seasons by means of the solstices and equinoxes. But for reckoning spans of time longer than a day and shorter than a year, the Moon was invaluable. If, for example, you knew from observation and memory that your major food-animal regularly migrated about four months after the winter solstice, it was far easier to count four Full Moons than 116 days. Knowledge such as this could make the difference between eating well and going hungry, between being clothed and shod and having a roof over your head, or enduring all sorts of discomfort. Ultimately, it might make the difference between living and dying. Similarly, knowing where and when to find plants for healing as well as for eating was vital, and information of this kind would be passed verbally from one generation to another.

The position of certain stars, or groups of stars, was another way to identify the time when a particular plant or animal might be found and in the clear skies of Africa, where the human race as we know it almost certainly emerged, they were easy to see. The connection between the appearance of this or that constellation in a particular part of the sky and recurring events on Earth would gradually become part of a clan's memory and of their survival strategy. And when some of the hunter-gatherers began to settle and grow crops, the same kind of observation helped them to predict rainfall and other crucial weather changes and decide on the best times to plant.

We have no way of knowing whether our far-off ancestors believed that the Sun, Moon and stars caused events on Earth, or whether they simply used the sky as clock and calendar.

All this is a long way from astrology. But certain fundamentals remain the same, namely, the position of the Sun, Moon and stars in relation to the timing of events on Earth. How such observations crystallised into what we would now recognise as astrology, nobody knows. Certainly a huge span of time separates those bones inscribed with the Moon's phases and the first-known evidence of astrology – millennia during which speech and writing evolved and people came to live in cities.

Drying aromatic plants to use as medicine is equally remote from modern aromatherapy, but the roots of our art lie in the earliest recognition by humans that certain plants had healing properties. From this grew the whole system of herbal medicine (which was virtually *all* of medicine for many thousands of years) and aromatherapy, which is a specialised branch of herbal medicine. It is no accident that these two arts, or sciences – for both disciplines embrace elements of science and of art – developed alongside each other in some of the earliest civilisations. When we look back across the great span of human history, we can see where there have been huge leaps, like the development of writing or the invention of the wheel, which have changed our history for ever, and periods of high civilisation that fostered the blossoming of many different disciplines. It often seems that several new ideas emerge at about the same time and that is certainly true of both medicine and astrology.

For example, the first evidence of a system that can be recognised as the beginning of what we now know as astrology comes from the Middle East from around 1650 BC but we must remember that before a system becomes codified it will have been in use for a long time, probably transmitted verbally before it was ever set down in writing. Stone tablets from before 2000 BC show that the Egyptians and Babylonians divided the sky into 36 sections of 10° each. By around 700 BC the Babylonians were using the Zodiac belt, though they included more constellations than we do now – it was another 200 years or more before this became the circle of 12 signs that we still use today, and Persian astronomers then began to organise the 12 unequal constellations into regular divisions of 30° each with which we still work. You will see that I use the term astronomer, for at that time (and for thousands of years thereafter) there was no distinction between astronomers and astrologers.

By this point in history we do know that people equated the planets with their gods and credited them with great powers, calling the planets 'rulers' or 'lords' of the various signs. Some of the terminology that they coined has survived in astrological use to the present day even though our belief systems are very different. Each successive civilisation adapted the names of the planets to those of their own pantheon, and it is those of the Olympian deities of classical Greece and Rome that have come down to us.

Not long after the time that the first modern Zodiac was developed, the great Hippocrates in Greece was teaching the connection between astrology and healing – though, as I pointed out above, before any body of knowledge is set down systematically, it will have been in use and evolving over a period of time. Hippocrates was what we would now call a holistic practitioner, considering the person as a whole, not just a collection of parts, emphasising the need to find the cause of any illness rather than treat the symptoms. He used and wrote about a large number of medicinal plants, including many that are part of modern aromatherapy such as coriander, cumin, fennel, frankincense, myrrh, roses and thyme. It is also clear from his writings that the relationship we now recognise between each sign of the Zodiac and certain parts of the body was already well-established in his day, for he advised against operating on parts of the body governed by the sign that the Moon was passing through. He also taught the theory of the four 'humours', choleric, sanguine, phlegmatic and melancholic, which remained the basis of medical treatment until well into the 17th century. The humours corresponded to the four elements as applied to the Zodiac signs: choleric to fire; sanguine to air; phlegmatic to water; and melancholic to earth.

The importance that Hippocrates attached to the link between astrology and healing can be seen from his statement that, 'Anyone who practises medicine without taking into consideration the movement of the stars is a fool.' Strong words indeed!

Generations of physicians drew on Hippocrates' teachings and some of them left important bodies of writing that both reflected his influence and built upon it, notably Dioscorides some 400 years after Hippocrates, and

Galen a generation later. Although Greek-born, they both worked in Rome and each left many volumes of writing on medicinal plants, including much astrological lore. When the Roman empire collapsed in the 5th century many of the Greek and Latin texts were taken to Alexandria and became part of the great medical library there. Many were later translated into Arabic, and it is to the Arabic civilisations from about the 6th century onwards that we owe the development of the complex system of astrology that we know today, as well as much medical knowledge. Inheriting the knowledge of earlier civilisations they built upon it, codified it and added to it.

Of all the great early astrologer-physicians, Abu 'Ali al-Husayn ibn 'Abd Allah ibn Sina, better known by the Latinised version of his name, Avicenna, is perhaps the most relevant to the story of aromatherapy, because he was for a long time credited with inventing the method for distilling essential oils from flowers. In fact, archeological finds show that rather primitive stills existed before his time, but he probably improved the technique by adding a cooling coil to the basic still. What is certain is that essential oils as we now know them – what Shakespeare later called 'all the perfumes of Arabia' – were first produced in Persia in Avicenna's time. He was born in 980 AD and became what we would now call a Renaissance man, skilled in a whole range of disciplines from Islamic law to poetry, via music, metaphysics, logic, mathematics and the natural sciences, as well as medicine and astronomy. He was an alchemist, too, and it is possible that he stumbled across the way to distil essential oils in the course of his alchemical experiments. He left major writings on all these subjects as well as the *Kitab ash-shifa* – *The Book of Healing* – which included not only descriptions of over 800 medicinal plants and their uses, but detailed instructions for various kinds of massage and manipulation and recommendations about detoxifying diets, any of which could be applied today.

So, the earliest forms of what we now know as astrology and aromatherapy all stemmed from the Middle East and the Mediterranean area, but that does not mean that parallel developments were not taking place in other parts of the world. The same significant date appears again, for both India and China had highly developed systems of plant medicine by 2000 BC and both developed their own systems of astrology. While Chinese astrology is based on somewhat different principles, the Indian vedic system has more in common with the Western tradition, perhaps as a result of contact with Greek culture in the 2nd century. Vedic astrology has always been an intrinsic part of Ayurvedic medicine and still is at the present day.

In north-western Europe the great megalithic monuments such as Stonehenge speak of a civilisation with highly developed mathematical and astronomical skills as much as 2,000 years before the first records of Babylonian astrology. Alas, in the absence of any written record, we have no way of knowing why these great monuments were built, but the colossal effort and organisation that went into their making shows just how important the observation of the heavens was for their builders and suggests that there was religious or ritual purpose for their construction. I find it hard to believe that people capable of such organisation, and the calculations that must have been needed to build such an accurate observatory (for that is what Stonehenge is, in essence), did not have a system of writing: probably they wrote on bark or similar fragile materials which would never survive several thousand years in a cold, wet climate.

It is clear that the structures were designed for viewing the sky, and particularly the Sun at the solstices but, just as we cannot know whether the earliest humans believed that the movement of the heavenly bodies influenced what happens here on Earth, we can only speculate as to why observing the midsummer sunrise was so important to the megalith-makers.

Whatever the purpose, clearly they had developed formidable skills in mathematics and astronomical observation and it seems probable that in the latter part of the Megalithic Age some of this knowledge filtered into the Mesopotamian area, where a dry climate has preserved the clay tablets and inscribed stones that tell us how traditional astrology began. In Egypt, papyruses with 'prescriptions' for herbal preparations have been well-preserved, so we can see how both astrology and medicine developed over a span of several thousand years into the organised methods that we find in the writings of Hippocrates, Galen and Avicenna.

It was such writings, particularly those of Hippocrates, Galen and Dioscorides, that became known in mediaeval Europe in Latin translations and formed the basis of much of the medical and astrological practice of the times. Some of the earliest European 'herbals' were little more than direct translations of the earlier texts, though later writers, such as Banckes and Gerard in England, Monardes, Mattioli and Charles de l'Ecluse on the continent of Europe, added their own observations. By this time, the application of astrology to medicine was one of its major uses, and physicians would base their treatment on an astrological assessment of both the patient and the time that they became ill. The greatest of the Elizabethan astrologers was John Dee who was consulted by Elizabeth I, most notably to decide upon the most propitious time for her coronation, and who warned her of the coming Armada (though as he was also a spy the latter observation may not have been entirely an astrological one!).

It was the astrologers of the next generation, though, who brought the practice of medical astrology to its peak but, ironically, also saw the seeds of its decline. Greatest among these was Nicholas Culpeper, to whom we owe much of our knowledge of the methods in use in 17th-century England. His great *Herbal* which assigns every plant described to a particular planet and contains much other astrological observation besides, has never been out of print, while *The Astrological Judgement of Disease*, which he published in 1655, remains the classic text on medical astrology, summing up the knowledge and methods that had evolved over the previous centuries and, indeed, millennia. He distinguished clearly between 'simples', that is herbal remedies that anybody could make for themselves, and 'chymical oils', which we now call essential oils. These were obtainable from apothecaries, and he stressed their considerable strength when compared to simples, and the need for knowledge and caution when using them.

The significance of Culpeper's books is that they were written in English, so that anybody who could read had access to clear information about medicinal plants, astrology and the practice of medicine. He also translated a large number of Latin medical texts, which brought him into direct conflict with the doctors who undoubtedly felt threatened at seeing that which had previously been their secret knowledge made available to all. The fact that Culpeper was not a doctor but an apothecary undoubtedly rubbed salt in the wound and the College of Physicians attacked him in various periodicals.

By now the doctors were beginning to use many more non-plant materials, some of them highly toxic, such as mercury for the treatment of syphilis which killed more people than the disease itself, and paying less attention to the astrological observations that earlier generations of doctors had used. As medicine became further removed from nature, so it became removed from the stars.

Astrology itself was also under attack from some quarters: Culpeper's great contemporary, William Lilly, was imprisoned on more than one occasion on charges of treason and indicted several more times for fortune-telling, in particular for predicting (accurately) the dates of the Great Plague and the Fire of London. Indeed, he was at one point suspected of having caused the fire in order to make his prediction come true.

By the end of the 17th century astrology as a whole and medical astrology in particular had largely fallen into disregard, in England at least, though it continued to be taught at some European universities. The climate of the time was not sympathetic to the complex, symbolic, mystical and often mystifying language of astrology that had developed in the mediaeval period, nor to its association with alchemy. The Age of Enlightenment was dawning, with its emphasis on clarity, logic and science. In medicine, the advance in surgical procedures and anatomical knowledge superseded the old doctrine of humours. Certainly the knowledge of herbal plants survived, but largely at the level of village wise-women, many of whom were persecuted on suspicion of being witches. Great thinkers were no longer drawn to the study of astrology, which was mostly looked down on as a form of superstition.

It wasn't until the end of the 18th century that the trend was reversed with the publication in England of Ebenezer Sibley's *New and Complete Illustration of the Occult Sciences* in 1790. Astrology began once again to engage serious thinkers with the emergence in the early 19th century of influential writers such as Richard Cross Smith who used the pen-name Raphael, and Richard Morrison, known as Zadkiel. These two founded the first organised astrology society in England, published specialised journals and lectured tirelessly. Later in the century Alan Leo introduced a spiritual dimension to astrology and founded the Astrological Lodge of the Theosophical Society. Medical astrology, though, had to wait until the latter part of the 20th century to experience a revival, largely by holistic practitioners.

The middle years of the century, from around 1930, saw a huge increase in the popularity of astrology, with the first newspaper columns appearing in England, while in France René-Maurice Gattefossé was sowing the seeds of what we now call aromatherapy. In fact he coined the word 'aromatherapie'. Working as a chemist in his family's cosmetic firm, which used essential oils extensively as perfuming agents, he became interested in their healing properties and began to seriously research them, eventually writing the very first book on aromatherapy as we now understand it. We should remember here, though, that essential oils and flower absolutes have an unbroken history of use in perfumery since the Middle Ages.

Another great pioneer in France was Marguerite Maury, who built on Gattefossé's work. She eventually settled in England, and it is to her early students that we owe the first flowering of the art in the English-speaking world. Dr Jean Valnet, a French army surgeon working in the 1950s, was another major figure in the development of the art.

The growth in popularity of holistic, 'alternative' therapies such as aromatherapy, herbalism and homoeopathy coincided very much with the discovery of Chiron. Indeed, Robert Tisserand's *Art of Aromatherapy* was first published in 1977, the same year that the asteroid was identified and includes attributions of each of the essential oils to a planet. In this Tisserand mainly follows the attributions given by Culpeper in the *Herbal* while some other authors have attempted new attributions, an area not without its problems, as you will see later in this book.

The other strand of 20th-century astrology which is of immense importance to our understanding of healing, regardless of the particular discipline involved, is the development of psychological astrology. Much of this has its origins in the work of Carl Jung, and has been further developed by such teachers and writers as Liz Greene and Howard Sasportas, among others. There has been a great shift in emphasis from prediction to the use of astrology as a way of understanding personality, and this is one of the main ways that holistic practitioners can draw on astrology. If we understand what 'makes somebody tick' we are better placed to help them.

Our understanding of how astrology 'works' has changed, too: few astrologers now regard the Sun, Moon and stars as the *cause* of events on Earth and in our lives, at least not in the gross sense that was implicit in the idea of 'Rulership' and planets as gods. Rather, it may be that the subtle energy, or 'prana' which pervades the entire universe may, in ways which we do not fully understand, carry an influence to us from even the most distant stars.

We have come a very long way since that adolescent sat on the hillside learning to observe the sky, and in the intervening millennia many came to believe that the heavenly bodies did, in fact, give rise to earthly events. But we can gain a deeper understanding of the value of astrology if we remember 'As above, so below' and see the sky as a mirror of life on Earth rather than as a controlling force. Again, the work of Carl Jung and his theory of synchronicity have been important in guiding us towards such an understanding.

I hope in this book to show how we can draw both on these relatively recent developments and on the knowledge of the relationship between plants, planets and people that has been distilled over the past 4000 years and more. We are fortunate, indeed privileged, to have access to the traditions of both East and West, and from this vantage point we can bring back together the two strands that were intertwined for so long but have largely been separated for the last three centuries.

I should emphasise that this is not a book about medical astrology. Medical astrology is based primarily on drawing up a chart for the moment a person first became ill, known as a Decumbiture Chart (from the Latin meaning 'to lie down'). If the time the illness began is not known, the time the person first consulted the practitioner is used instead. Further charts are used at critical times in the progress of the illness and decisions about what medicines or other procedures to use are based on them. All of this is a highly specialised field of study and presupposes a thorough grounding in ordinary astrology before even embarking on it.

What I hope to show, if you will follow me through these pages, is how aromatherapists and lay people using essential oils for themselves and their families or friends can draw on a much simpler understanding of astrology to guide them in the use of essential oils. Some of you may well want to go further and study medical astrology in depth but it is perfectly possible to enrich your understanding of aromatherapy simply with the information in this book and I wish you much joy in so doing.

★ HOW TO USE THIS BOOK

In writing this book I envisaged that possible readers might range all the way from professional aromatherapists who know little or nothing about astrology but would like to know more, to experienced astrologers who would like to learn about aromatherapy. I imagine, too, that the majority of you will fall somewhere between these two extremes, including aromatherapists with some knowledge of astrology, astrologers with more than an inkling about aromatherapy and people who use essential oils at home, have an interest in astrology and might be wishing to learn more about both!

Depending where you stand in this spectrum, you may want to use the book in slightly different ways:

IF YOU ARE A PROFESSIONAL AROMATHERAPIST

You can certainly skip the chapter introducing aromatherapy – there will be nothing in it that you do not know already. All the rest of the book will be relevant, with the chapters on the 12 signs of the Zodiac being particularly important. I hope that you will find that the astrological approach will enrich your practice.

IF YOU ARE AN EXPERIENCED ASTROLOGER

You will not want to read the chapter Finding Your Way Round a Birth Chart, which is very basic and intended for people with no experience at all of reading a chart. Do please, though, read all the other chapters, even though there will be much in them that you already know. Indeed, you are likely to know a lot more than is included here! However, the links between astrology and aromatherapy are explored in various ways throughout the book.

You will see that I have avoided the use of some common astrological terms, especially 'Ruler' and 'Rulership', preferring the expression 'planetary affinity' as coined by Jeff Mayo. I feel this better expresses our contemporary understanding, though I am aware that traditionalists may find it irksome, and to them I apologise.

EVERYBODY ELSE

Please read everything! If you use essential oils at home for yourself or your family and friends, I would ask you to pay special attention to the chapter on aromatherapy and, if possible, to follow this up by reading some of the other suggested books on the subject.

The essentials of aromatherapy

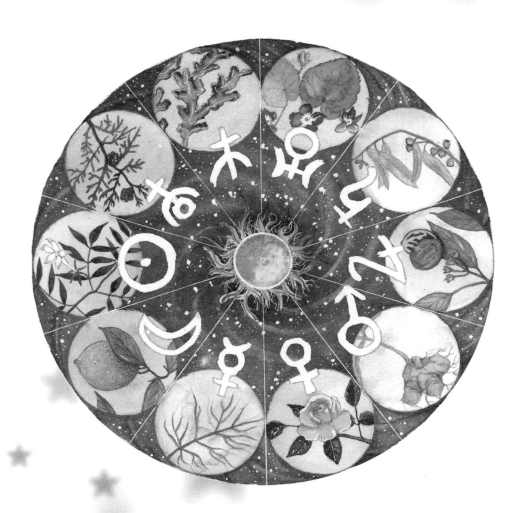

The essentials of aromatherapy

★ WHAT *IS* AROMATHERAPY?

Let's start by being sure that we are all talking about the same thing!

Strictly speaking, the word aromatherapy means the application of aromatic oils by a therapist, usually in the form of massage: in other words, 'aroma' plus 'therapy', though it is generally taken to mean the use of essential oils in many different contexts, many of which do not require the involvement of a therapist. Home use, in baths and room-perfuming for example, are valid examples of this, but the word is often misused to describe any kind of scented product, even those made with synthetic perfuming ingredients. Most of these are harmless – unless you have an allergic reaction to any of the ingredients – but they will not give you the beneficial results that the word 'aromatherapy' implies. Only genuine essential oils will do that, and in order to get the maximum benefit from them there are a few basic guidelines that need to be followed.

★ SAFETY IS PARAMOUNT

Essential oils are far more than mere perfumes. They are very highly concentrated materials, extracted from plants by distillation. Think of the difference between wine and spirits (which, of course, are also produced by distillation) and you will have an idea of the difference in potency between a herbal extract and an essential oil. Or, another way of looking at this: a colleague once calculated that three drops of Camomile oil contained as much of the active components of the plant as 75 gallons of Camomile tea!

They are very biologically active materials: if they were not, they would not have the healing effects that we expect from them, but biologically active materials also have potentially harmful effects. I once had a discussion with a medical doctor who refused to believe that aromatherapy was a valid form of alternative medicine, but when I mentioned an incident where somebody had made herself ill enough to be hospitalised after misusing essential oils he became really interested. If essential oils could make you ill, he reasoned, they must be pharmacologically active and could therefore make you well! That may be a very topsy-turvy kind of logic, but I cite it here because it illustrates the real potency of the oils.

This is not intended to deter you from using essential oils, but to emphasise that we need to treat them with respect and common sense. Simply follow a few basic rules and you can use them with complete confidence.

SOME SAFETY DO'S AND DON'TS

NEVER TAKE ESSENTIAL OILS BY MOUTH.

- Store essential oils in a safe place, out of reach of children.
- Always dilute essential oils before you use them.
- Keep essential oils away from the eyes, even when diluted.
- Do not use more than 6 drops of essential oil in the bath.
- Do not use essential oils if you are pregnant (or if the person you are working with is), without taking professional advice first.
- Take professional advice before using essential oils if you suffer from epilepsy, have high blood pressure or any diagnosed ailment.
- Do not use essential oils without professional advice if you are taking any prescribed medication: they may interact adversely.
- Be extra careful if using essential oils with babies and children or with frail, elderly people.
- Be extra careful with anybody who has sensitive skin: dilute well and try the mixture on a small area of skin first.
- Learn the list of dangerous oils, or refer to it if in doubt, especially when working with anybody in one of the groups listed above.

★ DILUTING ESSENTIAL OILS

Essential oils need to be diluted in a carrier oil before being applied to the skin, whether that is for skincare, massage, etc. Suitable carrier oils are grapeseed, soya, sunflower and other good-quality vegetable oils.

Almond oil is often used for facial massage and skincare, but is somewhat expensive if you want to do a full-body massage. Sesame-seed oil is an excellent carrier, and has the advantage that it washes out of clothes and towels easily. Always buy the best quality oil you can, cold-pressed if possible. Carrier oils have beneficial properties of their own, which may be lost if they are heat-processed. Vegetable oils oxidise easily, producing free radicals, when heated. Once you have bought them, store in the fridge which will keep them in good condition longer.

The usual dilution for massage is 3%. This is very easy to calculate – just add 3 drops of essential oil to each 5 ml measuring spoon of carrier oil. (Don't use an ordinary domestic teaspoon. They vary too much in size and most of them hold less than 5 ml.)

For a child, a frail elderly person or anybody with sensitive skin, use a 1.5% dilution – 3 drops to 10 ml of carrier oil. If in doubt about anybody's possible reaction to a particular oil, dilute well and try on a small area of skin before considering using it for massage, baths or skincare.

★ OILS IN THE BATH

When using essential oils in the bath – and this is probably the most common use of them by people other than trained therapists – just remember OIL AND WATER DON'T MIX! In other words, however much water there is in your bath it will not dilute the essential oil. The oil spreads out into an ultra-thin film which floats on top of the water. When you get into the bath, most of this film will cling to your skin and the heat of the water will help it to penetrate the skin so that you get the maximum benefit from it. A few oils which are perfectly safe when diluted in a carrier oil for massage can cause skin irritation when used in the bath. These include most of the spices and some citrus oils, particularly Orange and Grapefruit. Bergamot and Mandarin are safe, but remember not to use Bergamot in the bath in summer because it increases the skin's sensitivity to burning. Alternatively, you can dilute the essential oils in a carrier oil before adding them to the bath. This is also a good way to use them for people with dry skins.

Don't be tempted to use more than 6 drops of essential oil to each bath. This is an area where more is not necessarily better. Six drops may seem very little, but it is quite enough to have the effect you are hoping for, whether that is to soothe aching muscles, wake you up in the morning, help you sleep at night or a multitude of other purposes, depending on what oil(s) you choose. If you have sensitive skin, or you want to put oil in a child's bath, it is better to dissolve it in a little carrier oil first, then stir that into the bath. Babies' baths need extra care and we'll look at this next.

★ AROMATHERAPY FOR BABIES

Aromatherapy can be a wonderful help in dealing with the minor problems of infancy – teething, nappy rash, little skin irritations and so forth, as well as to help babies sleep peacefully, but it is important to be especially cautious both in the choice of oils and the dilutions and proportions. Some essential oils are really too powerful for use with babies, even when diluted. You will find a table of hazardous oils towards the end of this chapter.

Safe oils to use with even the youngest infants are Camomile, Lavender and Rose and of these Camomile is particularly well-suited to babies' needs as it calms and soothes inflamed cheeks during teething, sore bottoms and other minor skin irritations and upset tummies when rubbed gently into the baby's stomach.

Babies love being massaged, and you will often find baby-massage classes advertised in places where ante- and postnatal classes are held. Adding one single drop of Camomile, Lavender, Mandarin or Rose to 5 ml of almond or other carrier oil will make the massage even more beneficial. Lavender is particularly good at bed time, as it promotes calm sleep. You could also try putting a single drop on a cot sheet.

For babies' baths, again a single drop of essential oil is enough and you should always dilute it in a little carrier oil before stirring it into the water. Once babies are old enough, many parents like to take them into the bath with them, or pop them in with older brothers or sisters: great fun all round, but remember to dilute any oil you use in the bath to the proportions and quantities suitable for the youngest person involved, as described in the previous section.

★ OLDER CHILDREN

With children from, say, 3 years upwards, you can use 1.5% dilutions of oil for any application to the skin, and maybe 3 or 4 drops of oil in an adult-sized bath, but I would still recommend diluting the oil before adding to the water until children are 8 or 9 years old. You can widen the selection of oils used, too. From about 12 years' old onwards, you can use the directions for adult use, unless the child is very small for his or her age, or has very sensitive skin.

Aromatherapy can reduce the discomfort of all the common childhood illnesses, from coughs and colds and little tummy upsets to chickenpox and the other infectious diseases of childhood. Obviously you will consult a doctor or other professionally trained person for anything other than minor problems – I think mothers develop a sixth sense about this.

Always keep a bottle of Lavender oil handy for cuts, grazes, insect bites, rashes and minor burns. I have one in my kitchen, one in the bathroom and one in my handbag at all times, even though I'm a grandmother now, but it is even more important to be able to put your hand on a bottle when you have young children around you. For such day-to-day emergencies Lavender can be used undiluted – it is one of the few oils than can be safely used in this way.

Tea-Tree is another oil which is good for minor injuries. It is highly antiseptic, speeds healing and combats viral and fungal infections as well as bacteria, but it is a harsher oil than Lavender, and I would keep it for older children, and stay with Lavender for the under-fives.

There are many other ways in which essential oils can be used to smooth the passage through childhood for both parents and children, from banishing head lice to preventing travel sickness but there is not space here to cover them all in detail. May I suggest that you look in my earlier book, *Aromatherapy, an A-Z* for far more detail, or in Jane Dye's *Aromatherapy for Women and Children?*

★ AROMATHERAPY IN PREGNANCY AND CHILDBIRTH

I have been accused in the past of overcautiousness in writing about essential oils and pregnancy but, when dealing with the health of a mother and her unborn child, I would far rather be too careful than risk a tragedy. As a general rule, I would say DO NOT USE ESSENTIAL OILS IN THE FIRST THREE MONTHS OF PREGNANCY WITHOUT PROFESSIONAL ADVICE AND NOT AT ALL IF THERE IS A HISTORY OF MISCARRIAGE.

From the fourth month onwards, it is generally safe to use such gentle oils as Camomile and Lavender at 3% dilution, and the majority of other oils in 2% dilutions. However, there are some oils that can cause miscarriage or damage to either the mother or baby or both, and you will find these listed at the end of this section.

During labour, massage of the tummy, back or both with Lavender or Jasmine can ease discomfort and increase the efficiency of contractions. Gently massaging the tummy with either of these after the baby is born helps to expel the afterbirth. There are oils that help prevent stretch marks, and others to treat sore nipples – again, I would refer you to either my own or other books that deal more fully with this area.

★ ELDERLY PEOPLE

Aromatherapy can help ease the aches and pains that tend to afflict us more as we grow older, but in some cases it is wise to use caution when deciding on the choice of oils, the dilution and the method of use. In the Western world, the population as a whole is living longer and staying strong and healthy longer than even one generation ago, and most older people can use the same oils perfectly safely, in the same quantities and dilutions that are recommended for adults in general. It is only when somebody has become frail, in poor health, and who has perhaps lost a great deal of their former weight, that we need to take extra care. As a general rule, you should use only 2% or 1.5% dilutions, and dilute oils before adding them to the bath for a more delicate person. If somebody has become vague or forgetful, don't leave undiluted essential oils with them for their use, but make up diluted blends that they can use without any danger to themselves.

★ HAZARDOUS OILS

At the end of this section you will find a list of hazardous oils. Do, PLEASE, take careful note of it. You will see that some oils are listed under several categories: Not to be used in pregnancy; Skin irritant, etc. That is because they contain some powerful, naturally occurring chemicals which can have a damaging effect on more than one body system.

★ THE PRINCIPAL METHODS OF USE
MASSAGE

Massage is the most important way of using essential oils, and forms the core of aromatherapy. Many people find they can massage their family and friends effectively without training, but even intuitive masseurs can usually improve their skills with some tuition. There are innumerable massage courses on offer, long and short, and I would strongly urge you to take one if you want to massage your family or friends. This is something you really cannot learn from a book or a correspondence course, though the many excellent books that exist can help you remember the strokes you have been taught, and learn new strokes once you have acquired the basic skills.

AROMATIC BATHS

Aromatic baths are probably the most popular way of using essential oils at home. They demand no skill and don't require the presence of a therapist, although they are often 'prescribed' by professional aromatherapists too. This is a very versatile method and can be used to relax or stimulate, to ease muscular, arthritic and rheumatic pain, to ease depression or just for the sheer pleasure; in fact the uses are as varied as the essential oils at your disposal. The amount of oil to use has already been discussed among the safety factors, so simply remember to put the oil in the bath at the last minute, just before you step into the water, otherwise a large proportion of it will evaporate and your bathroom ceiling will get the treatment instead of you.

★ OTHER USES

Apart from massage and baths, you might wish to use essential oils in steam inhalations for colds, coughs and sinusitis, in vaporisers for room perfuming, as a personal perfume, to scent your laundry, and in skincare.

As a perfume, it is quite safe to put a single drop of oil directly on the skin, and a single drop is all you will need. None of the oils that are delightfully perfumed, such as Jasmine, Neroli, Rose, Sandalwood, etc. will irritate the skin, but check on skin-irritant oils in the lists at the end of this chapter, particularly if you have a sensitive skin or are prone to allergies. Be aware also that Angelica, Bergamot and one or two others can make the skin more sensitive to sunlight, so avoid putting them on any part of the body that will be exposed in summer time. I have known people suffer really bad burns through ignoring this advice, even when the oil was used as a perfume in the evening and they did not go out into the sun until the following day. Bergamot has a number of qualities that make it very suitable for summer time use: it is deodorant and refreshing, for example, so use it carefully, diluting to less than 2% before use. Remember that oil in the bath clings to the skin and is not diluted by the water (oil and water don't mix), so

31

put Bergamot in a carrier oil before adding to the bath water in summer time.

To scent laundry, you might put a few drops into rinsing water, or make your own perfumed drawer liners. Sprinkle a few drops of your chosen oil on some paper, roll it up and wrap in polythene for a week, then use it to line clothes drawers or those in which you keep the bed linen. I put bundles of dried Lavender in the airing cupboard. Many essential oils are effective insect deterrents, and a few drops in the wardrobe will keep moths away, Lavender and Cedarwood being among the most effective.

Room fragrancers are one of the most popular ways of using essential oils at home and they can do much more than just create a pleasant aroma. You might use them to help stop the spread of infection during epidemics, to keep insects out of your house, or to enhance a chosen mood. Ceramic burners that use a nightlight below a dish of water can be found more or less everywhere, but some of them are not well-designed and do, literally, 'burn' the essential oil, producing a nasty, tarry residue which is far from pleasant to smell and not at all therapeutic. Look for designs that a) leave enough space between the nightlight and the dish and, b) have a dish large enough to hold sufficient water for several hours' use without evaporating away completely. Alternatively, there are devices with a small electric element and a good-sized space for the water. They evaporate the essential oil slowly without overheating it and can be safely left on for long periods.

Steam inhalations are a very good way of clearing the nose and sinuses or soothing the throat and chest. You can put a single drop of essential oil in a bowl of very hot water and drape a towel over your head while you inhale the steam or, once again, you might like to invest in an electric 'facial sauna' if you think you are likely to use this method a lot.

Skincare is a huge area and, as with the treatment of babies and children, it is not possible to cover it in full here. You can find more detail in my earlier book, and in many other good aromatherapy and natural skincare books. In brief, facial massage with essential oils can be adapted to suit all skin types, depending on the choice of oil: Rose makes a luxurious facial oil, good for all skin types but especially older skin; Camomile or Rose are good for sensitive skins; Jasmine or Frankincense for mature skin; and Lavender, Bergamot or Tea-Tree for teenage oiliness. Geranium is a good oil for 'mixed' skin types, with oily areas in otherwise dry skin, as it balances the production of sebum – the natural oil in the skin.

★ BUYING ESSENTIAL OILS

The degree to which aromatherapy will produce the results that you expect depends a great deal on the quality of the essential oils you use. There are essential oils and 'aromatherapy' products on sale in a multitude of places now, from health-food shops and chemists to supermarkets and department stores. Unfortunately, not all of them are what they seem to be and, even where they are genuine essential oils, quality can vary a great deal. How do you find your way through this minefield?

First, price is a good guide: essential oils cost a lot to produce, some of them far more than others, because it takes a huge amount of plant material to make relatively little oil. The amount involved, and the ease or otherwise of extraction differs enormously from plant to plant, so good essential oils will vary widely in price across a range. If you see a range of oils that are all the same price, you can be certain that they are wholly or partly synthetic, or that they are diluted, or that they do not come from the plant named on the label! Look for brands that range from a few pounds for herbs such as Lavender or Rosemary through to precious flower oils such as Jasmine, Neroli or Rose which should cost up to twenty times as much, if not more! The latter are often sold in smaller quantities, or already diluted in a carrier to make them more accessible. Reputable brands will state on the label whether they are diluted. You will usually find authentic oils of this kind in health-food shops or from specialist mail-order suppliers.

Beware of oils described as 'nature-identical'...they aren't! Nothing is identical to nature except that which nature produces. There are some highly sophisticated methods of synthesising the more costly oils and the end result will do you no good at all, and just possibly some harm such as causing allergic skin reactions. Generally speaking, many of the oils in supermarket chains fall into that category. This is not the fault of the retailers but stems from far further back in the chain of supply. Let your nose be your guide: an authentic essential oil should smell like the plant whose name is on the label. Some of the cleverest synthetics get very close to the authentic aroma of a plant, but nothing can ever quite match the real thing.

Finally, try to buy organic or wild-grown oils whenever possible for your own sake and that of the planet.

Once you have got your beautiful oils, it is important to store them correctly. Properly stored, undiluted essential oils will keep in good condition for several years. Exposure to sunlight causes them to deteriorate quickly, and for that reason your oils will probably be packaged in brown or blue glass bottles when you buy them. But it is a good idea to also keep the bottles in a dark place such as inside a cupboard or in one of the many varieties of boxes that are made especially for this purpose. Air is another factor that spoils essential oils rapidly, so make sure you replace the caps on your bottles immediately after use and screw them back tightly. Extremes of temperature are not good for your oils either: don't keep them in the fridge, or near radiators, fireplaces, etc. A moderately cool place where the temperature does not vary too much is ideal.

While essential oils can safely be kept for several years, vegetable (carrier) oils oxidise and go rancid fairly quickly, so you should try not to store ready-mixed oils for too long as the carrier is likely to deteriorate and spoil the essential oil that is mixed with it. If you buy the costly floral oils in ready-diluted form, don't be tempted to keep them for more than a few months and, when you dilute oils yourself, only mix what you are likely to use immediately.

★ CONCLUSION

Finally, do consult a trained aromatherapist if you are in any doubt. Using essential oils from day to day to alleviate colds, 'flu, headaches, minor cuts and burns, general aches and pains and so forth is perfectly possible without professional training, but please do not be tempted to 'treat' beyond your ability. A trained therapist may also advise you to consult your GP, an osteopath, acupuncturist or other person with specialist training if he or she thinks you may need treatment that is outside the scope of aromatherapy. In such situations, you will often be able to use essential oils at home as a backup to whatever treatment is appropriate; here again, ask a fully-qualified aromatherapist for advice.

★ DANGEROUS OILS

These oils should not be used at all in aromatherapy. They are either toxic, capable of causing miscarriage or triggering an epileptic fit, or they can severely damage the skin. Some of them carry more than one of these risks.

ALMOND, BITTER	*Prunus amygdalis, var. amara*
ANISEED	*Pimpinella anisum*
ARNICA	*Arnica montana*
BOLDO LEAF	*Peumus boldus*
CALAMUS	*Acorus calamus*
CAMPHOR	*Cinnamomum camphora*
CASSIA	*Cinnamomum cassia*
CINNAMON BARK	*Cinnamomum zeylanicum*
COSTUS	*Saussurea lappa*
ELECAMPANE	*Inula helenium*
FENNEL (BITTER)	*Foeniculum vulgare*
HORSERADISH	*Cochlearia armorica*
JABORANDI LEAF	*Pilocarpus jaborandi*
MUGWORT (ARMOISE)	*Artemisia vulgaris*
MUSTARD	*Brassica nigra*

ORIGANUM	*Origanum vulgare*
ORIGANUM (SPANISH)	*Thymus capitatus*
PENNYROYAL (EUROPEAN)	*Mentha pulegium*
PENNYROYAL (N. AMERICAN)	*Hedeoma pulegioides*
PINE (DWARF)	*Pinus pumilio*
RUE	*Ruta graveolens*
SAGE	*Salvia officinalis*
SASSAFRAS	*Sassafras albidum*
SAVIN	*Juniperus sabina*
SAVORY (SUMMER)	*Satureia hortensis*
SAVORY (WINTER)	*Satureia montana*
TANSY	*Tanacetum vulgare*
THUJA (CEDARLEAF)	*Thuja occidentals*
THUJA PLICATA	*Thuja plicata*
WINTER GREEN	*Gaultheria procumbent*
WORM SEED	*Chenopodium anthelminticum*
WORMWOOD	*Artemisia absinthium*

★ OILS THAT SHOULD NOT BE USED DURING PREGNANCY

BASIL	*Ocimum basilicum*
BIRCH	*Betula alba, B. lenta, and B. alleghaniensis*
CEDARWOOD	*Cedrus atlanticus*
CLARY SAGE	*Salvia sclarea*
CYPRESS	*Cupressus sempervirens*
GERANIUM	*Pelargonium asperum*
HYSSOP	*Hyssopus officinalis*
JASMINE	*Jasminium officinale, J. grandiflora*
JUNIPER	*Juniperis communis*
MARJORAM	*Origanum majorana*

MYRRH	*Commiphora myrrha*
NUTMEG	*Myristica fragrans*
PEPPERMINT	*Mentha piperata*
ROSEMARY	*Rosmarinus officinalis*
TARRAGON	*Artemisia dranunculus*
THYME	*Thymus vulgaris*

(Plus SAGE and WORMWOOD which are on the 'Not to be used at all' list.)

★ OILS TO BE AVOIDED IN THE FIRST THREE MONTHS OF PREGNANCY

In addition to the oils listed above, the following should be avoided until the fourth month. If there is a history of miscarriage they should not be used at all. They can be used during the remainder of pregnancy, diluted to 1.5% or 2% for massage, or 3 to 4 drops added to a carrier oil for bathing.

CAMOMILE	*Anthemis nobilis, etc.*
LAVENDER	*Lavandula vera*
ROSE	*Rosa centifolia, v. damascena*

★ OILS THAT SHOULD NOT BE USED BY PEOPLE WITH EPILEPSY

FENNEL (SWEET)	*Foeniculum vulgare*
HYSSOP	*Hyssopus officinalis*
ROSEMARY	*Rosmarinus officinalis*

★ OILS WITH A RISK OF TOXICITY OR CHRONIC TOXICITY

These oils should be used cautiously and never for more than a few days at any one time.

BASIL	*Ocimum basilicum*
CEDARWOOD	*Cedrus atlanticus*
CINNAMON LEAF	*Cinnamomum zeylanicum*
EUCALYPTUS	*Eucalyptus globulus*
FENNEL (SWEET)	*Foeniculum vulgare*
HYSSOP	*Hyssopus officinalis*
LEMON	*Citrus limonum*
ORANGE	*Citrus aurantium*
NUTMEG	*Myristica fragrans*
THYME	*Thymus vulgaris*

★ SKIN IRRITANTS AND SKIN SENSITISERS

Always dilute these oils to 1% before use. Do not use on people with sensitive skin or known skin allergies.

ANGELICA	*Angelica archangelica*
BLACK PEPPER	*Piper nigra*
CINNAMON LEAF	*Cinnamomum zeylanicum*
CITRONELLA	*Cymbopogon nardus*
CLOVE (ALL PARTS)	*Eugenia carophyllata*
GINGER	*Zingiber officinalis*
LEMON	*Citrus limonum*
LEMONGRASS	*Cymbopogon citratus*
ORANGE	*Citrus aurantium*
NUTMEG	*Myristica fragrans*
PEPPERMINT	*Mentha piperata*

★ PHOTOSENSITISING OILS

These oils make the skin more liable to burning in sunlight. Do not use on areas of skin that will be exposed to the sun unless diluted to less than 2%.

ANGELICA	*Angelica archangelica*
BERGAMOT	*Citrus bergamia*
LEMON	*Citrus limonum*
ORANGE	*Citrus aurantium*

★ ESSENTIAL OILS AND THEIR MAIN PROPERTIES

ANGELICA	detoxifying, digestive tonic, diuretic, restorative
BASIL	antispasmodic, cephalic, digestive, stimulant, tonic
BAY LAUREL	analgesic, antiseptic, digestive, neurotonic
BENZOIN	antispasmodic, soothing, stimulant, warming
BERGAMOT	antidepressant, antiseptic, deodorant, urinary antiseptic
BIRCH	analgesic, detoxifying, diuretic
BLACK PEPPER	digestive, diuretic, rubefacient, stimulant
CAJEPUT	antibacterial, antiseptic
CALENDULA	antidepressant, skin-healing
CAMOMILES	anti-allergic, antidepressant, diuretic, sedative
CARAWAY	digestive, immuno-stimulant
CARDAMON	aphrodisiac, digestive, tonic, warming
CARROT	gall bladder and liver tonic, valuable in skincare
CEDARWOOD	antiseptic, astringent, stimulant, tonic

CELERY	detoxifying, digestive tonic, diuretic
CITRONELLA	antirheumatic, insect repellent
CLARY SAGE	antidepressant, antispasmodic, relaxing, sedative
CLOVE	analgesic, antiseptic, insect repellent
CORIANDER	analgesic, aphrodisiac, digestive tonic, warming
CUMIN	antispasmodic, digestive stimulant and tonic
CYPRESS	antispasmodic, astringent, deodorant, insect repellent
ELEMI	antiseptic, decongestant, tonic, stimulant
EUCALYPTUS	antiseptic, bactericidal, decongestant, diuretic
FENNEL	digestive, detoxifying, diuretic
FRANKINCENSE	calming, meditation aid, pulmonary antiseptic, tonic
GERANIUM	antidepressant, antiseptic, astringent, balancing
GINGER	antispasmodic, aphrodisiac, digestive, warming
GRAPEFRUIT	antiseptic, antidepressant, deodorant, diuretic
HELICHRYSUM	antidepressant, anti-inflammatory, antispasmodic
HYSSOP	antiseptic, mucolytic, reduces bruising
JASMINE	antidepressant, aphrodisiac, valuable in skincare
JUNIPER	antiseptic, astringent, detoxifying, diuretic

LAVENDER	analgesic, anti-inflammatory, antiseptic, antibacterial, antifungal, antiviral, decongestant, healing, sedative
LEMON	antiseptic, astringent, bactericidal, tonic
LEMONGRASS	antiseptic, bactericidal, insect repellent, tonic
MANDARIN	antidepressant, digestive, valuable in skincare
MARJORAM	analgesic, decongestant, rubefacient, sedative
MELISSA	anti-allergic, antidepressant, regulates menstrual cycle
MIMOSA	antidepressant, antiseptic, astringent, used in perfumery
MYRRH	astringent, expectorant, fungicidal, healing
MYRTLE	bactericidal, decongestant, sedative, urinary antiseptic
NEROLI	antidepressant, antispasmodic, aphrodisiac, sedative
NUTMEG	antiseptic, aphrodisiac, digestive, stimulant, tonic
ORANGE	antidepressant, astringent, digestive, sedative
PALMAROSA	antiseptic, digestive, balancing, hydrating,
PARSLEY	diuretic, tonic, vasoconstrictor
PATCHOULI	anti-inflammatory, antidepressant, antiseptic, tonic
PEPPERMINT	antiseptic, decongestant, digestive, warming

PETITGRAIN	antidepressant, balancing, mildly sedative
PINE	antiseptic, bactericidal, decongestant, stimulant, tonic
ROSE	antidepressant, aphrodisiac, menstrual regulator, perfume, tonic, uterine tonic, valuable in skincare
ROSEMARY	analgesic, antiseptic, cephalic, decongestant, stimulant, tonic
ROSEWOOD	analgesic, bactericidal, meditation aid, valuable in skincare
SANDALWOOD	antiseptic, aphrodisiac, bechic, meditation aid, perfume
SPIKENARD	antifungal, antiseptic, diuretic, warming, meditation aid
THYME	antiseptic, cephalic, decongestant, tonic, stimulant
TEA-TREE	antibacterial, antifungal, antiseptic, antiviral, cytophylactic, immuno-stimulant
VERBENA	digestive, insect repellent, sedative, tonic
VETIVERT	antidepressant, astringent, calming, immuno-stimulant, rubefacient
VIOLET LEAF	antiseptic, astringent, healing, perfume ingredient
YLANG-YLANG	antidepressant, aphrodisiac, balancing, hypotensive

Finding your way round
a birth chart

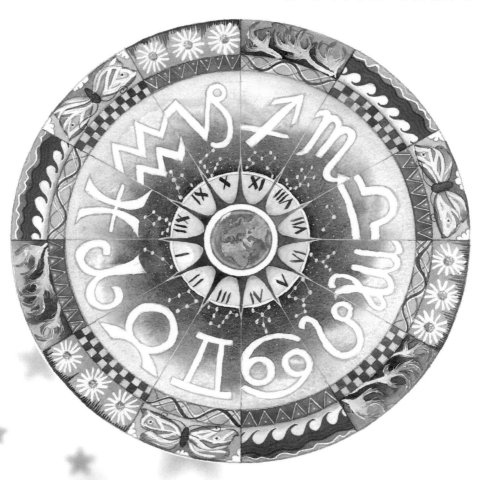

Finding your way round a birth chart

If you are a practising aromatherapist, or you use essential oils at home and would like to draw on astrology to help you, you may not be familiar with birth charts (or natal charts) and how to 'read' them. Charts are composed of a number of factors and, at first, they might look very confusing, so this chapter is intended to take you around the chart, examining each of these factors in turn. If you are already knowledgeable about astrology, you can skip this chapter completely!

First, let's consider what a natal chart is NOT: there is nothing sinister or magical about such a chart; it does not set out a person's future in an irrevocable manner or predetermine anything about their life or character. It is simply a map of the influences that were present when they were born.

One way to understand this is to liken the birth chart to the picture on a packet of seeds, i.e., it shows the *potential* of the person for whom it was calculated. How the person uses that potential depends on many factors, just as the seeds in a packet may grow into plants less or more like the picture, depending on soil, climate, location and whether the garden is well-tended, regularly weeded, etc. How that potential evolves will depend on both external influences, such as nurture and education, and internal factors, such as the level of consciousness of the individual and to what extent they are willing to take responsibility for their own actions.

A birth chart is made up of a number of components which interrelate, forming a synthesis which is UNIQUE TO THAT PERSON. No two birth charts are the same, with the very rare exception of twins born within a few minutes of each other. Even with twins there is usually enough time between the two births for the fastest-moving elements in the chart to have changed a little.

The main factors that make up a chart are: the Signs, Planets, Houses and Aspects. We also take into consideration the overall shape of the chart (i.e., how the Planets are distributed around the circle) and four key points on the circle, known as the Angles.

The chart itself is simply a diagram that shows the positions of the

Sun, Moon, Planets and Signs at the time of a person's birth, as seen from the place at which they were born. Imagine standing in a high place with an unobstructed view on a clear night. As you slowly turn around you can see the whole of the sky with the Moon and all the stars in a circle around you – that is exactly what your birth chart represents in diagrammatic form: the position of all the heavenly bodies at the time you were born, as seen from a certain spot on Earth. (If you were born in daylight hours, the Moon and all the stars were in exactly those places, even though they were not clearly visible at that time.)

Most often, the diagram is circular, though there are other formats: you may come across octagonal charts (popular in the United States) and in old books, or modern books that reproduce charts from much earlier sources, you may find square ones. The circular form is to my mind the best representation of the moment of birth, as we can imagine ourselves standing on the Earth in the centre of the chart surrounded by sky. It is also by far the simplest to read, as it is easy to mark on it the 360° that make up a circle and, as you will see in the next few pages, various ways of dividing up those degrees are an important part of understanding a chart.

★ SIGNS

To start with, the birth chart is divided into 12 equal sections of 30° each corresponding to one of the Signs: Aries, Taurus, Gemini, Cancer, Leo, Virgo, Libra, Scorpio, Sagittarius, Capricorn, Aquarius and Pisces, and these are identified by their symbols (or glyphs) written in the outer part of each section. The Signs are what the majority of people are familiar with in astrology, whether they have any other interest in the subject or not.

THE GLYPHS (or Symbols) FOR THE 12 SIGNS

♈	Aries	♎	Libra
♉	Taurus	♏	Scorpio
♊	Gemini	♐	Sagittarius
♋	Cancer	♑	Capricorn
♌	Leo	♒	Aquarius
♍	Virgo	♓	Pisces

The Signs in a natal chart tell us about the intrinsic nature of the individual, their true self, what 'makes them tick', how they are likely to behave in various circumstances, how they might relate to other people, and also something about their physical strengths and weaknesses. Because of this they are the first thing we will look at when using astrology to help us with aromatherapy, and they merit in-depth exploration, so we will consider each of them in detail in separate chapters. You may find that the information implicit in the Signs is all that you wish to incorporate into your use of essential oils or, once you feel confident in using that information, you may wish to explore further, in which case, the next feature of the chart to study is the Planets.

★ PLANETS

The positions of the Planets are also shown on a chart by means of their 'glyph' or symbol, usually placed near the outer edge of the circle and accompanied by figures that give their precise position in degrees and seconds.

THE GLYPHS (SYMBOLS) FOR THE PLANETS

☉	Sun	♃	Jupiter
☽	Moon	♄	Saturn
☿	Mercury	♅	Uranus
♀	Venus	♆	Neptune
♂	Mars	♇	Pluto
		⚷	Chiron

The Planets represent psychological archetypes. Every one of us embodies all these archetypes, or types of character, to a greater or lesser degree and the position of a Planet in the chart will often tell us which characteristics are likely to be strong in the individual and which will be less important. Each Planet has an affinity with a different Sign of the Zodiac, and understanding the nature of the Planet will expand our perception of that Sign and people born in it, so we will be exploring the Planets in depth later on.

Pay particular attention to the position of Chiron (⚷) in the chart as this can often give considerable insights into the origins of illness. Chiron represents wounding, but also tells us where healing can be experienced. The Sign in which Chiron falls might tell you something about vulnerable parts of the body, while the House where Chiron is found will suggest the

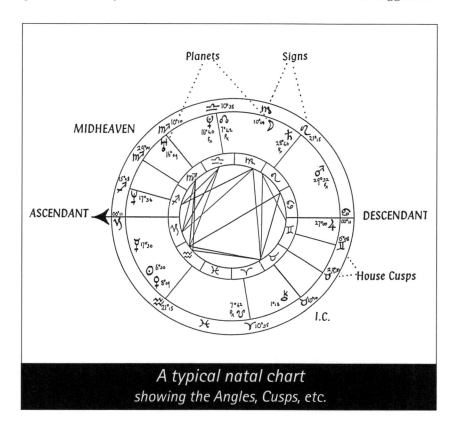

A typical natal chart
showing the Angles, Cusps, etc.

area of life experience that may have given rise to the problem. If you can see that Chiron is conjunct to a Planet, or makes a hard aspect to a Planet, consider the nature of the Planet involved as it can tell you a great deal about the roots of illness.

Planets also have an affinity with various plants (and therefore the essential oils distilled from them) and these Planet/plant connections are a major element in considering aromatherapy from an astrological point of view so, once again, these connections will have a whole chapter devoted to them.

★ HOUSES

The next component of a birth chart that we need to consider is the Houses. If you look at the circle of a birth chart you will see that, as well as being divided into sections corresponding to the 12 Signs, it is also divided by lines, rather like slices cut into a cake, and these slices correspond to the 12 Houses. The two sets of divisions do not necessarily correspond with each other. A House seldom begins at exactly the same point as a Sign, and may occupy less or more than 30°. (We'll look at why, later.)

Each of the Houses represents an area of experience, such as work, play, relationships, health, talents, friends and so on, and a person's experiences in these different areas can have a significant impact on their health, so an understanding of the Houses can be valuable when planning aromatherapy treatments. As with the Signs and Planets, we'll look at the Houses in detail in a separate section of this book and examine the different areas of life experience that each House represents.

★ ASPECTS

The word 'Aspects' is used in astrology to describe angular relationships between the Planets as they appear in the chart. They are shown on natal charts by lines connecting the Planets involved.

Thousands of years of observation suggests that when Planets are separated by a certain number of degrees they relate to each other easily or less easily, and taking note of the relationships between the various Planets in an individual chart tells us something about how that individual is likely to experience and express the character of the Planets involved.

The word 'Aspect' is connected with the idea of looking, and it's helpful to think of Aspects in terms of how the Planets 'look at' each other. In this book we will only consider the five major Aspects: the Trine, Sextile, Square, Opposition and Conjunction. There are a number of others, but these five will serve us well in the present context, and if you are curious about astrology you may want to explore the others via books or training courses.

The **Trine** symbol △ is an Aspect in which two Planets are 120° apart, or a Planet is 120° apart from one of the Angles, such as the Ascendant, for example. This is generally considered the 'easiest' and most harmonious of all Aspects, where energy can flow freely between the Planets involved. For example, a Trine between the Sun and the Moon would suggest that the individual will be able to integrate their masculine and feminine sides without difficulty, while a Trine between the Moon and the I.C. (Imum Coeli) tells us that this person will probably attach great importance to the home, family life and the experience of parenting. Where there are a great many Trines in a chart though, particularly if they are not balanced by some more difficult Aspects, it can suggest that the individual is at risk of being too easy-going, that life is not presenting them with enough challenges.

The **Sextile** symbol ✳ is an Aspect where two Planets (or a Planet and an Angle) are separated by 60°. It is similar in nature to the Trine, but tends to have a more practical application. It often indicates a talent. For example, a Sextile between the Moon and the Midheaven could indicate that the individual would be successful at using their homemaking or mothering skills professionally – maybe they will run a crèche, or become an interior designer.

Opposition ☍ is the name of the Aspect where two factors are 180° apart, i.e., they lie directly opposite each other on the circle of the chart. We can best understand the nature of an Opposition by going back to the idea of how Planets look at each other. In Opposition, they metaphorically cannot avoid each other's eye. Oppositions often point to a tug-of-war situation in a person's life: Saturn opposite Uranus implies a conflict between authority and freedom, for example.

The **Square** symbol □ is, of course, the 90° angle and is another challenging Aspect. Where we see a Square, there are usually issues that need to be addressed. If the person concerned ignores these issues, there will often be stress that may be the underlying cause of physical illness. An example might be a Square between Saturn and Jupiter: Jupiter encourages our excesses, Saturn asks us to be moderate. The challenge here is to find the middle way: too much excess can lead to many different forms of disease, too much moderation can lead to self-denial, meanness, repression or frustration.

Finally, the **Conjunction** symbol ☌. This is where two Planets are extremely close to each other, or a Planet is very close to an Angle. We consider two points to be in Conjunction when they are less than 8° apart and we may think of them as merging their identities. For example, a Mars/Mercury Conjunction indicates somebody who will bring great energy to mental tasks, a Neptune/Venus Conjunction shows somebody who is likely to be highly intuitive, spiritual and artistic but who at the same time may allow themselves to be deluded in romantic matters.

In some charts you will find Aspects involving more than two Planets. The **Grand Trine** involves three Planets, each 120° from the next, and appears on the chart as an equilateral triangle. Energy can flow harmoniously between all three, in the same way as a simple Trine, and the person with a Grand Trine in their chart will generally find satisfaction in the areas suggested by the position of the Planets involved and may often be talented in those areas, though there is a risk of laziness or a *laissez-faire* attitude, simply *because* everything is so easy.

The **Grand Cross** on the other hand is an extremely challenging configuration, made up of two Oppositions at right angles to each other, so that each of the four bodies involved is also linked by a Square. As you may imagine, a Grand Cross in the chart indicates areas of struggle in an individual's life, but this is not necessarily all bad. People who face up to the challenges involved and deal with them positively grow in the process and are generally very strong in character.

The **T-Square** consists of an Opposition in which the two Planets are also in Square to a third. On the chart it looks like half of a Grand Cross, and presents something of the same challenge, but in a less extreme form. It gives us an idea of where the challenges in life will be, and the focus needed to overcome them. People who meet these challenges successfully usually show great determination and the ability to get things done.

Most charts show a combination of 'hard' and 'soft' Aspects, which work together with the Sun, Moon, Ascendant and other factors to build our characters.

If a natal chart is drawn in colour, there will probably be a key to tell you which colour represents which aspect: the most usual system is to use green for Trines, blue for Sextiles, red for Squares and purple for Oppositions, though some people use red for both Squares and Oppositions. If the chart is drawn in monochrome, the Aspect Lines may be variously shown as dots, dashes and unbroken lines, identified by their symbols.

A certain amount of leeway is allowed in calculating Aspects: a few degrees on either side of those I have quoted are permissible.

★ THE ANGLES

The Angles are four particularly sensitive and significant points on the chart, which are best understood as two opposite and complementary pairs.

The **Ascendant** marks the precise moment of birth. It represents the Sign that was rising at that time, in other words, the group of stars that were physically coming up over the Eastern horizon at that moment, as viewed from the place where the person concerned was born. (You may sometimes hear the Ascendant referred to as the Rising Sign.) You will find it marked on the left-hand side of a chart, in a position roughly corresponding to 9.00 on a clock face, and often emphasised by an arrow, or by a thick or coloured line. It marks the beginning of the first House, which is concerned with our Self, our primary experience of the world and how we present ourselves to the world.

The Ascendant tells us about a person's outward personality, how they engage with the world, how they present themselves to others. This may be quite different from the deep, inner self represented by the Sun in the chart, but it will usually colour the first impression we receive of that person.

Perhaps you have met somebody whose Sun Sign is, say, Taurus, but their behaviour, the impression you have of them, is so unlike what you know about Taurus you think, I'd never have believed s/he was a Taurean. Almost certainly this person has a Sign on their Ascendant which is very different from Taurus in its manifestation. Dig deep, though, and you will find the Taurean underneath. The difference between the character of a person's Sun and that of their Rising Sign can lead to conflict and unhappiness if the individual is unable to integrate the various parts of their personality but, equally, it is part of what makes each one of us a complex, interesting individual.

Whereas, for example, everybody born between 21st March and 20th April in any year will have their Sun in Aries, their Ascendant may fall in any one of the 12 Signs, depending on the time and place of their birth, as each of the Signs will be rising on the horizon in the course of every 24 hours. If you were born around dawn, your Ascendant will be the same as your Sun Sign. The Ascendant then changes as each of the Signs will then come up over the horizon in the course of 24 hours. Some take longer than others to traverse the horizon, but on average the Ascendant changes roughly every two hours.

When considering aromatherapy treatment, bear in mind the Ascendant if you know it. It may give you additional information or suggest a further selection of oils in addition to what you can deduce from the Sun Sign. Some astrologers consider that the Ascendant is a good indicator of physical appearance, particularly of the face, and of bodily strengths and weaknesses, while others think (as I do) that the Sun Sign is more reliable. Knowing the Ascendant, though, can sometimes be useful when an individual displays strengths or weaknesses that cannot be related to their Sun Sign. Also note which planet is associated with the Sign on the Ascendant: this will be one of the most important Planets in the chart – the astrologers of old called it 'The Lord of the Chart'.

The **Descendant** is exactly opposite the Ascendant, 180° around the circle, and is shown as a slightly heavier line on the right-hand side of the circle – around 3 o'clock. It represents, literally, the Sign that was setting on the Western horizon at the moment of birth and, figuratively, the beginning of the seventh House, which is concerned with partnerships of all kinds. These may be business or professional partnerships, marriage or long-term relationships or even creative partnerships such as singer/accompanist, playwright/producer, etc. You can see how these two Angles complement each other, the Ascendant being about Self and the Descendant about Others.

The other two Angles are the **I.C.** or **Imum Coeli**, sometimes called the Nadir. This is the lowest point on the chart and in most systems of chart calculation corresponds to the beginning of the fourth House, symbolising the home and the experience of mothering, the place where we feel safest, that we retreat to when we feel threatened.

Opposite the I.C. is the last of these special points, the **M.C.**, or **Midheaven**, at the highest point of the chart. This represents our role in the outside world, and usually marks the beginning of the 10th House, to do with career or status in the world, how others see us. In many people's lives there are difficulties involving the opposing pull between home and career, our private life and how other people see us – these are I.C./M.C. issues in astrological terms.

★ THE NODES

These are two points on the natal chart which mark points where the Moon's path crosses the path of the Sun. They signify past and future influences, the South Node signifying where we are coming from and the North Node where we are going to. Some astrologers think of the South Node in terms of early infancy and antenatal experiences, while others see it as an indication of past-life influences. Which school of thought you choose to follow will depend on your personal belief system – though they are not mutually exclusive and you might find both approaches relevant in considering an individual and their chart.

There is general agreement that the North Node indicates the goal to be aimed at in life: look at the House and the Sign that the North Node falls in and then consider the person involved. Are they pursuing a goal in life that is in keeping with what the North Node suggests? Much stress, dissatisfaction and depression stems from following a life path that is not in accordance with one's true nature.

(NOTE: Some astrologers, and some astrology software programs only mark the North Node on a chart but it is easy to find the position of the South Node as it is always directly opposite the North Node, or 180° round the circle.)

★ THE SHAPE OF THE CHART

I've left this till last, but it is really the first thing we see, the first impression we get when we look at a chart initially, and first impressions do count. This concerns where and how the Planets are distributed around the chart: are they all bunched together, are they more spread out, etc? For example, if you see that the majority of Planets are located in the lower half of the chart, you can be fairly sure that this person is very focused on home, their personal issues and their private life, whereas if the Planets are mostly in the upper half of the chart the converse is true: the emphasis will be more on life in the outer world, career, status and interaction with other people.

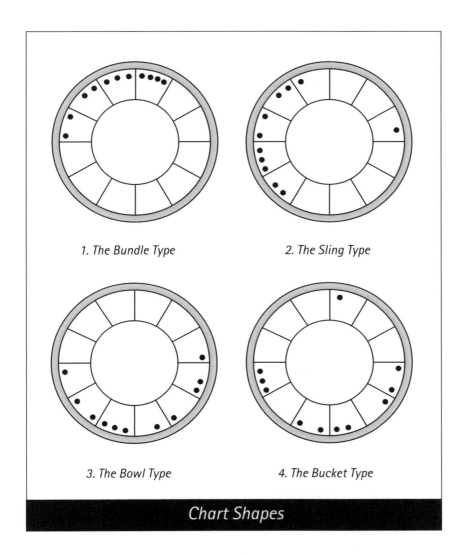

1. The Bundle Type

2. The Sling Type

3. The Bowl Type

4. The Bucket Type

Chart Shapes

1. The Bundle Type

All the Planets fall within approximately one-third of the chart. People with this chart pattern tend to concentrate all their energies into a narrow range of activities or have highly specialised interests. The leading Planet in the group (reading in a clockwise direction) gives an idea of the nature of those interests. This pattern is fairly uncommon.

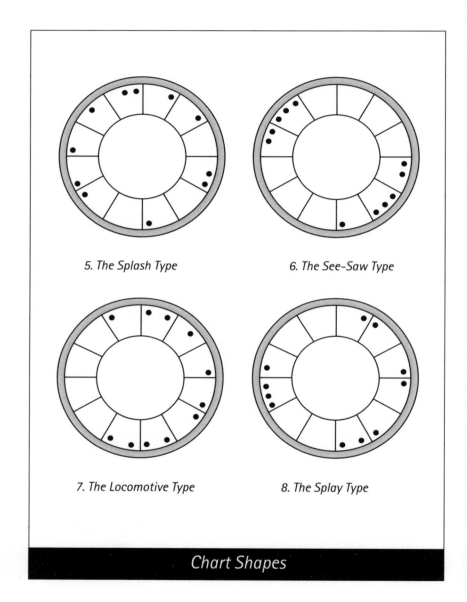

5. The Splash Type   6. The See-Saw Type

7. The Locomotive Type   8. The Splay Type

Chart Shapes

2. The Sling Type

This shape is like a bundle, but with one Planet outside the main group. People with this type of chart can be highly focused, but are able to communicate their special interests to the outside world.

3. The Bowl Type

Where all the Planets fall in one half of the chart, energies are concentrated in half of that individual's potential experience of life. The position of the 'bowl', in the upper or lower half or the left or right side of the chart, will indicate which experiences these are and, once again, the leading Planet gives the main impetus.

4. The Bucket Type

This is like the Bowl except that there is a single Planet separate from the concentrated group and, as with the Sling type, this Planet serves as a way to move energy out into a wider sphere.

5. The Splash Type

Where the Planets are spaced more or less evenly around the chart, the individual is likely to have far more varied interests and experiences. This is the most frequently seen type of chart.

6. The See-Saw Type

Where the Planets are concentrated in two groups, more or less opposite each other, the individual may feel pulled in opposing directions and will need to find a point of balance.

7. The Locomotive Type

Where the Planets are all located in two-thirds of the chart, the empty one-third represents an area of challenge. People with such charts are often very self-motivated. As with the Bundle type, the leading Planet 'drives' the locomotive.

8. The Splay Type

If the Planets are arranged in what appear to be random groups and do not conform to any of the above patterns the person is likely to be highly individual, possibly non-conformist.

★ CONCLUSION

In the following pages we will explore some of these components of the natal chart in more detail, namely, the Signs, Planets and Houses. The Sun Signs will be our first guides in discovering how astrology can help us in the practice of aromatherapy. Once you are familiar with the Signs, and are able to incorporate your knowledge of them into the way you use essential oils, you may feel that this is as far as you wish to explore. If so, you will already have a valuable and practical tool at your disposal. I hope, though, that you will want to explore further and add to your repertoire an understanding of the Planets and Houses and how they interact with the Signs.

Astrological Aromatherapy

Sun signs and aromatherapy

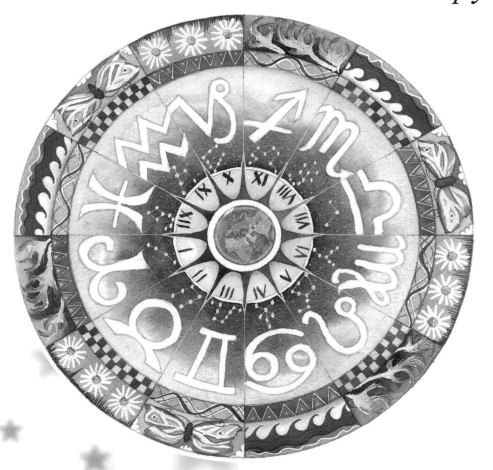

Sun signs and aromatherapy

Even if you know nothing else about astrology you probably know your Sun sign. This is sometimes known as the Star sign, or Birth sign.

When we say, "I'm an Aries, she's a Leo, he's a Scorpio," we are talking about the position of the Sun in that person's birth chart, which is expressed in terms of which sign of the Zodiac the Sun was in when they were born. This is where most people's acquaintance with astrology begins, with their 'stars' in a newspaper or magazine. Some never go any further. Of course, there is a great, great deal more to astrology than this, and we will explore much of it later in this book, but in terms of working with aromatherapy and astrology together, understanding Sun signs is a valid starting point. Even with no other knowledge of astrology they can help us in our choice of essential oils and their application.

Each sign is characterised by certain traits of psychology and personality and there is also a well-recognised correlation between the signs and different areas of the body, which may help us to identify an individual's physical strengths and weaknesses. You will find these correlations in the chapters on the individual signs. Each Sun sign also has affinities with a particular planet and plants can be associated with certain planets, too. Putting these various pieces of information together is a valuable tool for deciding on the most appropriate treatment.

Most people know their own Sun sign – even those who profess not to be interested in astrology! – but if they don't, or if you prefer not to ask this, you can easily identify it once you know their birthday. If you are working with a friend or relative you obviously know this already and if you are a practising therapist this is a routine question which you will ask at the first consultation. Do be careful, though, if the birthday is very near the beginning or end of the dates given for their sign: because human calendars are never in 100% agreement with the actual movement of heavenly bodies, so in some years the Sun moves into a different sign a day earlier or later than the commonly accepted date. If in doubt, consult a professional astrologer or check the Sun's position in an ephemeris (a table showing the positions of the planets day by day). If you have astrology software, that's another way to find out the position of the Sun, Moon or any planet on a given date.

Once you know the correct Sun sign, you immediately have access to some insights on personality, vulnerable areas of the body, the type of problems most likely to affect this person, and an indication of which oil, or combination of oils, is most likely to help. You can start straight away with your treatment plan, armed with knowledge that might otherwise only emerge slowly, over the course of a number of treatments...or not at all, if the person chooses not to disclose it. Indeed, they may not even be consciously aware of some of the factors that their Sun sign reveals.

When choosing oils for yourself, your Sun sign can be a valuable guide, too. It can be quite difficult to select oils for personal use, particularly if this is for treatment as opposed to simple enjoyment, as we can't always be sufficiently objective. In the absence of a therapist, I always feel that referring to the astrological factors is like having a second opinion.

In fact, I would seriously suggest to anybody wishing to bring astrology into their practice of aromatherapy that they start by working with the signs alone and bring other factors, such as the planets, houses, aspects, etc., into play once they have thoroughly familiarised themselves with the fundamentals.

So, we will begin by studying the Sun signs. These are groups of stars that form shapes in the sky which ancient civilisations identified as animals (mostly) or other shapes, and gave names to: the Ram, Bull, Twins, Crab, Lion, Young Woman, Scales, Scorpion, Archer, Goat, Water Carrier and Fishes. It is interesting that widely different civilisations gave similar names to these constellations.

There are many other named constellations such as the Plough, Orion, the Dragon, etc., but in astrology we are only concerned with these 12 because they lie along the Zodiac, a pathway or 'belt' around the Earth through which the Sun appears to travel, taking one year to move through all 12 Signs. (I shall not go into the question of the possible 13th sign here – you might like to explore it independently.)

Today, these constellations are no longer in the same positions they occupied when long-ago observers named them, due to a phenomenon know as the Precession of the Equinoxes. Put simply, star time is not the same as our earthly measurement of time and over a period of many thousands of years the two have got out of step. This does not alter the effectiveness of the system. Rather, it emphasises that the signs have more to do with understanding the kind of energy prevailing at different times of the year than to any influence the stars might exert. The spring equinox marks the first day of Aries, although the Sun is no longer in the sign of Aries at that time, but the kind of energy that is prevalent around the equinox has a very Arien quality and the same holds true of all the other signs.

Of course we know, as our distant ancestors did not, that the Sun does not move around the Earth, passing through this belt in its progress. Rather, the constellations themselves form a backdrop against which we view the sky as the Earth travels in her orbit, but this does not change the significance of the signs. The *nature of the energy* that prevails at the times we associate with each sign is the same whether we understand the structure of the solar system or not.

The myths surrounding the creatures after which the signs are named help us to understand the character of the signs and we will explore these in the section about each sign. Myths arise out of the needs and instincts of humanity and they embody deep truths in allegorical form. The great psychotherapist, Carl Jung, understood this very profoundly and incorporated it in his writing and teaching which forms the basis of modern psychological astrology as well as the more classical forms of psychoanalysis. Our experience of life and the world around us may be different, more complex, than that of the societies in which the myths originated, but these stories, and those concerning the ancient gods after whom the planets are named, still hold profound significance for us. They are far more than naive fairy tales and embody fundamental truths, particularly about the human psyche. When we talk about an Oedipus complex, or describe somebody as jovial, saturnine, narcissistic or Junoesque, we are drawing on classical mythology whether we are aware of it or not.

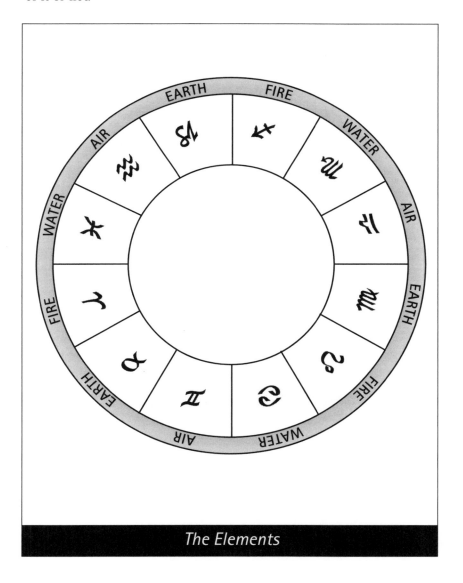

The Elements

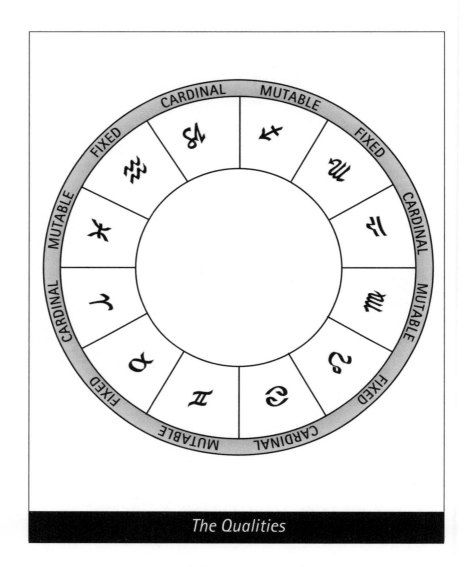

The Qualities

Our understanding of each sign is further helped by the fact that each one is described in terms of an Element: Fire, Earth, Air or Water, and a Quality: Cardinal, Fixed or Mutable. (You may find the elements described in astrology books as the Triplicity: a division of the Zodiac into groups of three, and the Qualities as the Quadruplicity: a division of the Zodiac into groups of four.)

The three Fire signs are: Aries, Leo and Sagittarius; Earth: Taurus, Virgo and Capricorn; Air: Gemini, Libra and Aquarius; and Water: Cancer, Scorpio and Pisces. Fire-sign people are usually passionate, eager, sometimes impatient, possibly quick-tempered, while Earth signs are more phlegmatic, practical, fond of material things, sometimes stubborn. People born in Air signs tend to be quick-witted, emotionally detached, more interested in things of the mind, while Water-sign people are archetypically deep, emotional, imaginative, sometimes rather hard to pin down.

The Qualities are perhaps not quite so easy to classify: Cardinal signs signify the beginning of something (each of them marks the beginning of a new quarter of the chart). The Cardinal signs are Aries, Cancer, Libra and Capricorn, and people with any of these Sun signs tend to be inquisitive, keen to push forward and get things done. The Fixed signs are Taurus, Leo, Scorpio and Aquarius. These signs tend to resist change. What the Cardinal signs have set in motion, they will implement and preserve. The Mutable signs of Gemini, Virgo, Sagittarius and Pisces are, as their name implies, more adaptable, more willing to change.

An analogy which I have found very helpful in understanding the Qualities was used by an astrologer friend who likened them to somebody travelling. When you first arrive in a new place it is exciting although unfamiliar, you are eager to explore, to discover all that the place has to offer, try everything out – this is Cardinal. When you have been there some time the place feels familiar, you feel comfortable and at home there, maybe you even think you'd like to settle down and spend the rest of your life there – this is the Fixed quality. Finally, when you know the place really thoroughly you begin to think you'd like to explore further afield, you are ready to move on – this is what Mutable is like.

When we put all these factors together we have a complex and sensitive tool for understanding the psychology of people, including ourselves, and when we know what 'makes someone tick' we are better equipped to help them with their problems, physical or otherwise. You will find in the following chapters a certain emphasis on stress, and under-standing the root causes of stress. This is because a great deal of physical problems have their origin in mental/emotional stresses, and because astrology is a valuable tool for exploring those origins. There are, as you will see, certain correlations between the 12 signs and various areas of the body, but I believe that it is the insights into an individual's psyche that are likely to be the biggest benefit you will derive from uniting aromatherapy with astrology.

It is worth remembering, too, that a person can be very strongly Libran (for example) even if they do not have their natal Sun in Libra, if they have a Libra Ascendant or Moon or several planets grouped together in the same sign. If you feel that somebody's nature is very different from what their Sun sign would suggest, this may be the case. Essential oils suggested for that sign may be more appropriate than those for their Sun sign but you would need to know their whole natal chart to be certain. However, we can safely start by looking at the 12 signs on the understanding that *most* people will be most strongly influenced by the position of the Sun in their chart.

★ SIGNATURE OILS

Throughout the chapters on the 12 signs, you will find references to 'Signature Oils'. What is a signature oil? It is an essential oil which, in some way, reflects the character of a particular sign of the Zodiac.

It is not necessarily the most therapeutically useful oil for people born under that sign, though it may well be. It is not always the favourite oil of such people: it often is, but I have come across people who detest the signature oil for their sign, even one or two who have an allergic reaction to it!

From the astrological point of view, a signature oil may not be what one would traditionally expect in relation to that sign, in that it is not associated with the corresponding planet...though here, yet again, that is sometimes the case. If we examine the sequence of elements in the Zodiac, a correlation can be seen. For example, there is a warming quality to all the oils associated with Fire signs, and a cooling one to those that mirror the Water signs, but there is no single, theoretical basis to the idea of signature oils.

It is simply something that I arrived at intuitively after many decades of working with essential oils. To test my idea, I began asking everybody I knew about their use of essential oils, which was their favourite, which did they use most often, etc. Their answers were enough to suggest that there was validity in my ideas. But in order to test it more rigorously, I devised a questionnaire which has been completed anonymously by a wide cross-section of people, both lay users of oils and trained aromatherapists and some fascinating facts have emerged. For example, when non-aromatherapists completed a questionnaire about their use of essential oils and their preferences, a little under half named the signature oil for their Sun sign as their 'favourite' and a further 20% named the oil that corresponded to their Ascendant or Moon. It was necessary to take into consideration that the 'favourite' oils named were often the more aesthetically pleasing fragrances, such as Jasmine, Neroli, Rose and Sandalwood as well as the ubiquitous Lavender. However, when practising aromatherapists completed a similar question about their use of oils for their clients, the therapeutic value of the oil was obviously more important than the fragrance. Here the correspondence between the clients' Sun signs and the oils that were found most valuable in treatment rose to well over 50%, and again where the Ascendant or Moon sign was known these corresponded to the oils used in another 15% of cases.

When talking with couples, the favoured oil was frequently the signature oil of the individual's partner: in other words, there would seem to be a relationship between some quality which attracted them to the oil and what attracted them in a person. (None of these people knew the purpose behind my questions nor what the 'right' answer might be, though where I was able to ask them personally I did enlighten them afterwards.) I was amused to note that both Gemini and Libra people tended to name two oils in the same breath, or say, "Well, it depends…"

Once we have identified an individual's signature oil, what do we *do* with it? Possibly nothing! Just knowing it may be all that is needed. I hope that, for those who are very familiar with essential oils but less familiar with astrology, these oils will help them understand something of the nature of the signs and that the converse will be true for astrologers who would like to know more about essential oils.

However, in choosing essential oils for treatment it helps to bear the signature oil in mind, perhaps in a blend with other oils that meet their immediate needs. I believe that the therapeutic function of the signature oil is *to bring a person back to their self.* This may be physically, when they have been depleted by illness, overwork, travel, etc., mentally or emotionally when they are under stress, or spiritually, if that is their desire.

You will find a description of each signature oil in the section relating to the Sun signs as the Sun in astrology symbolises the true Self, but if you know the individual's Moon and Ascendant, consider the appropriate oils for them, too. You may be able to employ all three in a blend, though this will depend on the person's birth chart – if these three chart factors throw up three oils that would not blend well from the aesthetic or therapeutic point of view it would be useless to put them together. Signature oils are not meant to be used as a rigid system or to replace a proper knowledge of aromatherapy, but to be one more tool in the aromatherapist's repertoire.

Astrological Aromatherapy

Aries

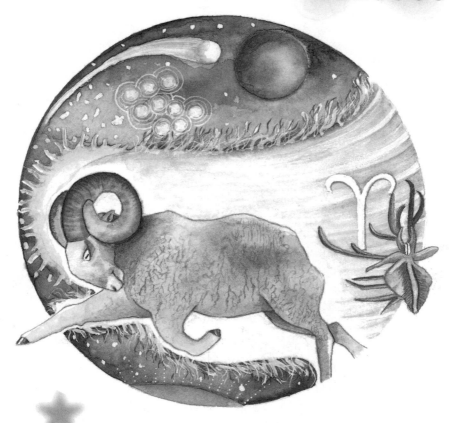

Ram's horns, sprouting seed or gushing fountain,

Zodiac's fiery firstborn rushes forth,

Questing, meeting, tasting life,

Pathfinder, mouldbreaker.

Aries

Aries Symbol: Υ

21st March - 20th April

Planet: *Mars*

Element: *Fire*

Quality: *Cardinal*

Signature Oil: *Rosemary*

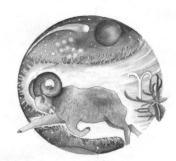

The Zodiac year begins with the sign of Aries, the Ram. The Sun enters this sign at the spring equinox in the Northern Hemisphere, a time of new energy and the beginning of the 'natural' year, as opposed to the calendar year. In fact, pre-Roman calendars did begin at the spring equinox.

A number of early myths depict a ram as a saviour or rescuer: the Greek story of Athamas and Phrixus, where Zeus sends a golden ram to rescue the boy who is about to be killed by his father, is almost identical to the Old Testament tale of Abraham and Isaac. Possibly the Zodiacal Ram was considered as a saviour because the advent of spring rescued people from the hardships of winter. It is worth remembering here that winter, long, long before electric lighting, central heating, canned foods and home freezers, was a time of real hardship and deprivation so the arrival of spring meant infinitely more to these people than a mere improvement in the weather.

So, Aries reflects in many ways the character of spring. Its symbol, though usually understood to represent the Ram's horns, can also be seen as the seedling plant bursting through the soil. This kind of energy finds an echo in the Aries character: Ariens generally are eager for new experiences, often pioneers or leaders in their field, or opening up new fields entirely. Here again the old stories tell us something about the nature of the sign. The tale of Jason and the Argonauts is an Arien myth: the hero sets out on a quest for the Golden Fleece, which came from that same Ram that saved Phrixus, surviving many dangers and eventually succeeding. Aries loves adventure and will exhibit great courage when necessary, though this can sometimes show itself as foolhardiness and lack of judgement. Another possible downside of the Arien character is a tendency to overpower those around them. This is usually unintentional, due rather to their innate enthusiasm and energy, but in extreme cases may become a desire to dominate rather than lead.

Possibly the people who helped Jason in his task can be seen as symbolising the fact that Ariens are far better at initiating things than following them through to completion unless there are other elements in the chart (such as the Moon or Ascendant in an Earth sign) that help them to manage the repetitive day-to-day chores. They are usually decisive, both mentally and in movement but above all they are 'doers' and anything that prevents them being active can quickly lead to frustration and sometimes depression. So when an Aries is in need of help from aromatherapy it will often be for these reasons. The planet Mars, with which Aries is associated, is characterised by driving energy and Ariens will often push themselves to the limit – and beyond – resulting in exhaustion or burn-out.

This sign is related to the head and the Arien will often be prone to headaches, migraine, catarrh, sinusitis and other problems affecting the head. Fortunately, these are all conditions that respond very well to aromatherapy treatments. Because this sign tends to be impetuous, accidents in general and especially accidents to the head are not uncommon. If these are minor, such as bruising or slight abrasions, you may well be able to help, but obviously more serious head accidents need expert treatment.

The planet associated with Aries, as we have seen, is fiery Mars, and when an Arien is physically depleted it is often valuable to look to Mars plants in order to restore some of their innate energy. Mars plants (and essential oils, of course) are typically the fiery ones such as Black Pepper or Ginger. Conversely, when an Aries person is agitated, stressed or frustrated, the soothing oils ruled by Venus will be more appropriate. Supreme among Venus oils is Rose, with Geranium a close second.

The influence of fiery Mars makes Ariens vulnerable to fevers and inflammations, and for these cooling, Moon-related oils such as Camomile or Melissa are invaluable.

For the depression that sometimes assails the Arien I have found that Sun oils are more helpful than the fiery Mars oils, as they bring in the Fire element in a gentler way. Traditionally, the Sun is recognised as the ruler of the resins: Benzoin, Frankincense and Myrrh, all of which have warming properties allied to their calming, meditative effects. Bergamot and Orange – the 'happy oils' – belong to the Sun too, and they are, of course, the supreme antidepressants.

★ SIGNATURE OIL

Rosemary is the signature oil for this sign: it is a warming, stimulating oil with an incisive, 'no-nonsense' aroma that is very like the directness of the Arien. In blends, very little goes a long way: more than a tiny proportion will dominate any other oil that is mixed with it. The Rosemary bush grows fast and vigorously and is one of the first of the aromatic shrubs to flower in spring. The oil is excellent for treating the headaches, sinusitis and catarrh that often plague Aries people. It is wonderfully restorative when they have pushed themselves to the limit, and beyond, tonifying weary muscles and refreshing a tired mind. It is a herb of the Sun, but Culpeper, who tends to be more precise than most in his attributions, says that it is "ruled by the Sun in Aries".

Taurus

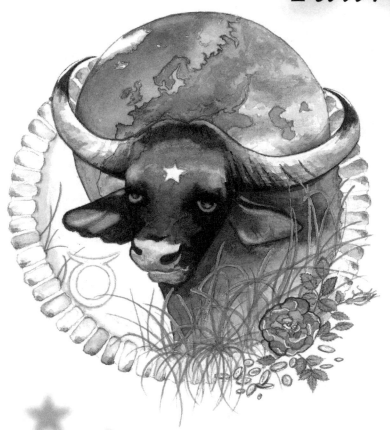

The Bull conserves, maintains, defends,

Savouring his treasures and his loves,

Digs deep into mother Earth

And stands, and stays and holds.

Taurus

Taurus Symbol: ♉
21st April – 21st May
Planet: *Venus*
Element: *Earth*
Quality: *Fixed*
Signature Oil: *Rose*

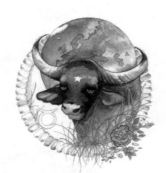

Where Aries pioneers, Taurus consolidates. The cautious Bull values its assets and, indeed, in earlier times cattle were one of the major assets that people valued. The herd represented the milk and meat, butter and cheese that fed the community; clothing, footwear and shelter (in the form of tents, yurts and the like) came from their leather and there was wealth in their value as barter. The bull was vital to the survival of the herd and therefore the community, for without him the cows could not be impregnated. So the bull became a fertility symbol. Both bull gods and cow goddesses are often found in ancient cultures from Babylon to Egypt and from Persia to Rome, where the worship of Mithras, the bull slayer, involved the ritual sacrifice of a bull to ensure fertility.

May Day, the present-day name for the ancient feast of Beltane which marked the end of spring and the beginning of summer, falls during the time of Taurus and, in a few places, dancing round the phallic maypole reminds us that this was originally a time to celebrate fertility as well as a great fire festival. In Celtic rites, cattle were driven between two fires at Beltane. In 17th-century England, the Puritans banned all May Day celebrations because of the sexual licence involved in the celebrations.

All of this is relevant to our understanding of Taurus. Taureans have a very shrewd appreciation of assets and values, both material belongings and intangible assets such as talents and abilities, but they also love all the fleshly pleasures: food, wine...and sex! So it is no surprise that the planet with which Taurus has affinity is Venus, the Goddess of Love and patron of beauty and the arts. Taureans are often very talented people with a keen aesthetic sense: they appreciate fine clothes, comfort and tasteful surroundings and are often prominent in such professions as fashion or interior design. Beauty therapists often have Taurus prominent in their charts too.

Music is another art associated with this sign and many Taurean people are either music lovers or performers. Taurus' emphasis on the throat often gives a beautiful voice, but as well as singers many famous dancers are Taureans too.

Lest we should think that Taureans are exclusively materialistic, with their emphasis on value, security and sensuous pleasure, many of them express the earthiness of the sign through a deep love of the planet Earth. This may take the form of concern for the environment and involvement in environmental causes, through gardening or, going right back to the roots of Taurus, through agriculture and animal husbandry.

Taureans have the patience, determination and tenacity to stick at a task or project and see it through to completion. The same qualities are found in their relationships with people: they are loyal and steadfast, forming life-long friendships and making great efforts to maintain their marriages or relationships. If taken to excess, though, these characteristics can have a negative effect. Tenacity can become stubbornness, fidelity can turn to jealousy, and the Taurean will sometimes stick with a situation when it would be in their best interest to let go.

Over-indulgence in some of the good things they appreciate can be a Taurean weakness, so you may find Taureans looking for help with digestive difficulties, weight problems or cellulite. On the credit side, they will love the sensuous delight of fine aromas and are likely to respond very well to therapeutic massage though they also love to be pampered and will often book a massage simply for relaxation.

It's worth noticing, in passing, that the very characteristics that make Taurus people such appreciative receivers of aromatherapy also make them very good aromatherapists! They are extremely sensitive to the beautiful aromas of the oils, and tend to have a real talent for giving massage. In my experience as a teacher of aromatherapy I certainly found a higher-than-average proportion of Taureans among the most able students.

Taurus governs the neck and shoulders and, when giving massage to Taurean people, you will often find that these areas are stiff and tense, as they tend to store up their worries here. There is often a tendency to throat infections, too, and sometimes to thyroid deficiency.

It goes without saying that Taureans will love all the luxurious oils ruled by Venus, such as Rose, Geranium, Sandalwood and Ylang-Ylang. But Earth signs tend to be slow-moving, both physically and metaphorically and Taurus, being of the Fixed quality shows this more than the other two Earth signs. Put those two words together – Fixed Earth – and you will get the feeling of this side of the Taurean character. Depending on how this manifests you may find the fiery Martian oils valuable, or it may be more appropriate to use oils associated with the speedy planet, Mercury. Of these, Caraway is a good digestive aid and Fennel is the 'shifter', the detoxifier par excellence, ideal for eliminating the results of Taurean overindulgence.

★ SIGNATURE OIL

The signature oil of Taurus is Rose, sacred to Venus and the epitome of beauty, both visually and in its aroma. It embodies the Taurean love of luxury and earthly delights, whether used as a perfume, a bath oil or for massage – the latter being particularly suited to this very physical sign. Its connection with Venus reminds us that it is a superb aphrodisiac, well suited to the Taurean delight in earthy pleasures. In fact, you can even eat Roses, candied, made into Turkish Delight or as Rosewater sprinkled on a desert, and if you have never tasted Rose wine you have missed a rare delicacy. It is among the most costly of essential oils, reminding us that Taurus is a shrewd judge of value. The more robust side of Taurus is echoed in the fact that Rose bushes will grow in virtually any soil and are extremely tenacious, surviving conditions that would kill a weaker plant.

Gemini

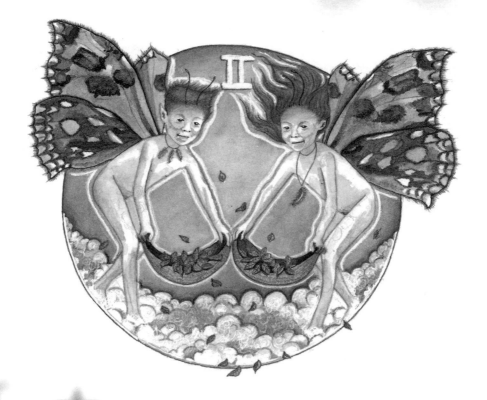

Mercury's airy Twins,

Sunshine and shadow, laughter and pain,

Quicksilver clever, never ever

The same two days together.

Gemini

Gemini Symbol: ♊

22nd May – 22nd June

Planet: *Mercury*

Element: *Air*

Quality: *Mutable*

Signature Oil: *Basil*

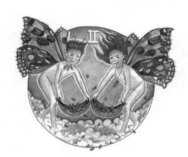

The sign of Gemini, the Twins, lies between spring and summer, and some people see that as the significance of the sign. The Roman poet, Manilius, said, "One of the twin brothers brings blossom and springtime, the other brings on thirsting summer," but there are twin myths far older, and of far deeper significance than that. They often tell of the division of day from night, or the Earth from the sky and frequently symbolise the struggle between good and evil. Early Indian astrologers saw this sign as the Divine Lovers, symbolising male and female. The two major stars in the constellation of Gemini, representing the Twin's heads, are named for Castor and Pollux, the twin sons of Leda. Castor was a mortal, the son of Leda's husband, but Pollux was fathered by Zeus in the form of a swan, and therefore immortal, so we have another example of two opposites linked. (Referring back to Aries and the story of Jason and the Golden Fleece, Castor and Pollux were among the crew of the Argo, who supported Jason on his quest.)

Gemini has obvious affinities with Mercury, the planet of communication and understanding, and Gemini people tend to have very lively minds: quick, versatile, enquiring, sociable, chatty, they may have a higher-than-average IQ and are often brilliant speakers or writers. Many Geminis are drawn to careers in the media, IT or other forms of communication. They often have a great deal of charm and may be flirtatious, though in a completely innocent way. Their natural curiosity may lead them to flit from one interest to another, change careers, homes or marriage partners more often than some people would find comfortable or, conversely, take on too many commitments at once. When a Gemini seeks help from aromatherapy it is likely to be because of mental stresses resulting from trying to keep too many balls in the air, and 'mental' is the key word here, though the stresses will usually manifest physically. The Gemini mind is restless and these people very often find it difficult to 'switch off' and relax. Consequently insomnia can become a major problem, especially for the elderly Gemini.

With so much emphasis on the mind, some Geminis become great worriers. At its most extreme, this can manifest as neurosis beyond the scope of aromatherapy. There is greater risk of this if the Air element is weak in the natal chart.

Some Geminis live in their heads to the detriment of their bodies: skipping meals or eating junk food, not getting enough sleep and failing to take exercise because they are totally preoccupied with their mental processes.

Every sign holds the potential for negative development, as we have seen, and occasionally you may see the versatility of Gemini developed to such a degree that they appear to have almost two personalities – a Jeckyll and Hyde situation. Another possibility is that charming, clever, sociable Geminis cut themselves off psychologically from their 'shadow' side; they refuse to acknowledge their own dark thoughts or negative behaviour. Here again we are talking about situations beyond the scope of aromatherapy, but an understanding of the natal chart may sometimes help us to steer people in the direction of counselling or psychotherapy.

Physically, Gemini has affinities with the arms, the lungs and also the central nervous system. Bearing in mind that the most important part of the central nervous system is the brain, and that this system is the major way in which the brain communicates with the body, can help us to understand the symbolism of how the different signs are associated with the various parts of the body. The arms, too, are important for communication: we write with our hands, whether it be with a pen or, more often now, via a keyboard. Rheumatic or arthritic pains in the arms have long been regarded as typically Geminian problems, but nowadays these avid communicators are likely to spend long hours at their computers to express their lively thoughts or exchange ideas via the internet, so look out for bursitis and repetitive strain injury. We use our arms and hands, too, to communicate when we punctuate or emphasise our speech with gesture, and to express ourselves when speech is not enough, or is impossible: think of international sign language, of how we resort to mime in a foreign country and how, in moments of high emotion, we may use a hug to show our sympathy more effectively than words.

The association of Gemini with the lungs is partly through the element of Air, which rules this sign and fills our lungs, and partly because the lungs, too, enable communication – we need air in order to speak, as well as for the vital processes of life. Geminis are susceptible to bronchitis or asthma, particularly in childhood and there is often a tendency to breathe too shallowly, which can contribute to feelings of nervousness or even panic.

Gemini's planet, Mercury, is also associated with a great many plants from which essential oils are obtained, including Lavender, all of which can be very useful in treating Gemini problems. Basil, the signature oil, is useful in treating lung infections and asthma as well as helping with mental alertness when the usually sharp Gemini is feeling tired or foggy. Thyme or Peppermint have the same stimulating effect while Lavender, on the other hand, can slow down the overactive mind and ground Geminis in their bodies.

★ SIGNATURE OIL

Gemini's signature oil, as we have seen, is Basil, a very mentally stimulating oil, akin to this sign's predominantly mental nature. The plant itself is very variable – another Gemini trait – with leaves that may be light or dark green, large or small, smooth or hairy. The aroma of the oil is very true to that of the plant and is often associated with holidays, Mediterranean food, pleasure and relaxation, reflecting the charming, sociable side of Gemini. But Basil also holds a hint of the darker side of the Twins: in folklore it has long been associated with Scorpio, as if to remind us that there is far greater depth to Gemini than is often acknowledged.

Cancer

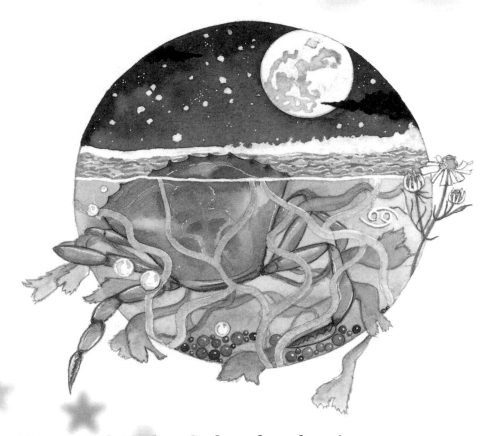

Moon-ruled Mother-Crab, soft and caring,

Hiding her hurt in armoured shell,

Makes her home deep, so deep

In ocean's watery breast.

Cancer

Cancer Symbol: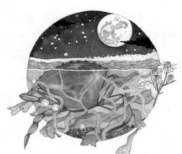
23rd June – 23rd July
Planet: *The Moon*
Element: *Water*
Quality: *Cardinal*
Signature Oil: *Blue Camomile*

The Sun enters the sign of Cancer at the time of the summer solstice, the longest day of the year in the Northern Hemisphere, which is one of the great fire festivals and has been so in many diverse civilisations. This may seem at first to sit oddly with the fact that Cancer is a Water sign but if we look a little deeper we find that the fires mark the *end* of the lengthening days and, as the days begin to draw in, we look inwards, to home and family, and this is the realm of Cancer.

The sign is associated with the Moon which was the Great Mother in many creation myths, and in astrology symbolises emotions, the unconscious and also motherhood and mothering. All of these are very important in understanding the intrinsic nature of the Cancerian. They are often deeply emotional people, though they may not find it easy to express their feelings, hiding inside their 'shell' like the Crab for whom the sign is named. Within the shell, though, they are often extremely vulnerable. This shell is vital for the Cancerian's emotional well-being, separating them from the overwhelming ocean of emotions outside, which might otherwise become more than they could manage.

The shell is the Crab's home, and the home is important to Cancerians, not only as the physical place where they feel safe, but as the place where the family belongs. Mothering and parenthood are central to Cancerians, both male and female, and they care deeply for their children. If they are separated from their children for any reason, whether it be due to the breakup of a relationship, or geographical distance when the children grow up and go their own way, they feel the loss acutely. Conversely, they need to feel loved and nurtured by their own mothers, and if this nurture has been lacking in childhood, the hurt can persist throughout adult life. They may expect their partners to take a 'mothering' role in their lives.

Physically, Cancer correlates with the stomach and pancreas and digestive problems of emotional origin are very common in this sign. Cancerians are often secret worriers, and tend not discuss their concerns with anybody else so this may be another cause of digestive problems. Cancer is also linked to the breasts (but please note that being born in the sign of Cancer does NOT mean that one is more likely to develop the illness of the same name).

It is easy to see the connection between the breasts and stomach and the strong Cancerian theme of mothering: mother nourishes the child first from her breasts, and later with solid food, and there are powerful emotional correlations between the physical act of feeding and the larger issues of nurture and mothering. How often in adult life do we express love via food? We give chocolates to our sweethearts, or take them out for a special dinner, or cook a favourite meal for our adult children when they come home to visit. Of course, Cancerians aren't the only people to do this, but they will have a greater tendency to show affection in this way than some of the other signs.

Emotionally, the Cancerian may be liable to strong mood swings and, in a few extreme cases, to paranoia.

Because they develop such a protective shell, Cancerians may not be the easiest people to help with aromatherapy. They may be somewhat resistant to massage, lying rigid on the couch and taking a very long time to relax although, ironically, they will benefit from the relaxation and therapeutic touch more than most. It may initially be easier to gain their confidence by giving them essential oils ready-diluted to use at home which will meet their need for privacy, or by suggesting oils for the bath; this way they can feel nurtured in the very element in which they are at home.

Unlike some signs, Cancerians seldom need the oils which are governed by their own planet. Moon-ruled oils are, in general, cooling and Cancer in trouble – whether physically or emotionally – is most often in need of warming. Just as the Moon reflects the Sun's light, Cancer people often benefit most from oils that are ruled by the Sun. The warm and cosseting character of Benzoin and the sunny citrus oils, such as Bergamot, Orange or Tangerine can all help lift Cancer out of the watery depths.

★ SIGNATURE OIL

Everything about Blue Camomile finds an echo in the character of Cancer. It is above all the 'Mothering' oil: calming and soothing, gentle enough to be used for even the youngest infants and appropriate for so many of the troubles of early childhood. Remembering that Cancer is associated with the stomach, we find that Camomile is used to ease stomach cramps, colitis, gastritis and diarrhoea, especially if they have their root in stress or anxiety.

All the Camomiles are similar in their action but Blue Camomile is the one most appropriate to Cancer because its colour evokes the Water element and the ocean that is the Crab's natural home.

Astrological Aromatherapy

Leo

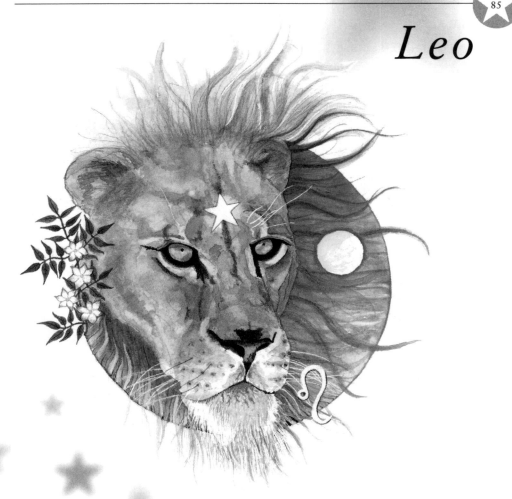

At Summer's height, the Lion-King
Basks in Sol's heat, reflects his fire,
Letting the rays ignite his ardent heart,
Lover, parent, artist, player.

Leo

Leo Symbol: ♌

24th July – 23rd August

Planet: *Sun*

Element: *Fire*

Quality: *Fixed*

Signature Oil: *Jasmine*

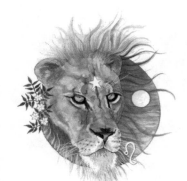

Having completed the cycle of the elements with Cancer, we start again in Fire with Leo, but the Fire energy here is subtly different from that of Aries. Where Aries is pioneering, pushing forward, with Leo there is a feeling of having arrived. (This illustrates well the difference between the Cardinal and Fixed qualities.) Where Aries typifies everything we associate with spring time, Leo is high summer, when the Sun is high overhead and we can bask in its warmth.

Leo just loves to bask in other people's attention, to be centre stage, hardly surprising as its traditional 'ruler' is the Sun, the centre of our solar system. Even shy, introverted Leos need recognition, perhaps even more than the extrovert ones.

The constellation was called a lion by civilisations from Babylon to India. In Egypt, it was connected with Sekhmet, the lion-headed goddess and in this story she is the mother of the Sun. The Greeks and Romans associated it with the story of Hercules and the Nemean Lion, which is almost identical to that of Samson and the Lion, that is, a human hero killing a lion with his bare hands. This association with heroes persists in our understanding of the Leo character.

Leo is traditionally the sign of kings and, by extension, to political leaders. It is also the sign of the performer: the actor, musician, dancer, pop star, though you will find an abundance of Leos in all the creative professions. Leo people suffer if their creativity is blocked, perhaps by the demands of parenthood or the need to earn a living in a routine job. Having an affinity with the fifth house, this is also the sign of FUN, of hobbies and leisure pursuits and Leo people do need to take adequate time for recreation.

When life circumstances seem to deny them that centre-stage position, or the freedom to express their creativity or, indeed, to play, Leos may suffer from depression – it is as if a dark cloud has covered the face of the Sun. This may be short-lived, but in some cases it becomes prolonged and extreme. Even in depression, though, Leo likes to be the centre of attention: where other depressed people might retreat into silence (think of Cancer, the Crab who will hide in its protective shell) they want to talk about their misery. The Bach Flower Remedy, Heather, relates to exactly this psychological state. Fortunately, we have a wide repertoire of antidepressant oils to choose from, many of which – Bergamot and Orange most noticeably – are associated with the Sun, so particularly appropriate for helping Leo people. Even so, it may be that your Leo friend or client will want to talk more than they will want a massage or advice about oils for home use! Their signature oil, Jasmine, of which I will say more later, is of major importance. If the depression is more than a short-term problem it would be responsible to suggest counselling or psychotherapy, but be warned: you may find Leos very resistant to such suggestions, sometimes to the extent of discontinuing their aromatherapy treatment. Great tact is needed here.

Physically, Leo correlates with the heart and the arterial circulation – you can see a clear analogy here between the Sun at the centre of the planets and the heart at the centre of the physical body. When the Leo person does not take enough time for recreation or creative activities, high blood pressure, palpitations or more serious heart problems are possible. So helping these people to truly relax may be the most important facet of aromatherapy treatment for them. Co-operation with a medical doctor is particularly important if there appears to be any hint of serious heart problems. We should also remember that 'heart' can be read as relating to the emotions, particularly to 'affairs of the heart'. Leos feel any disappointment in love very keenly and can be completely overwhelmed by the breakup of a relationship. This may trigger the kind of annihilating depression described earlier. It is no accident that a lion's family is called his pride and Leos are inordinately proud of their partners and offspring. They will often choose partners who are very good-looking, who they enjoy showing off in public. Similarly, they will show off their children and their children's achievements, whether it is their first word or high grades at school.

When working with Leo people, avoid the oils ruled by Mars: they can be overheating. Choose calming, comforting oils from among those which have affinities with Venus or the Moon such as Camomile or Melissa. Ylang-Ylang, a Venus oil, is particularly appropriate if palpitations are experienced. When a Leo person needs a warming oil, for example if they are depressed or physically depleted, choose a Sun oil such as those already mentioned, Benzoin or Myrrh.

★ SIGNATURE OIL

Only Jasmine is good enough for Leo! Just as the Lion is considered King of the Beasts, so Jasmine has long been called the King of Oils (Rose being the Queen). This is an oil that is redolent of sunshine, the plant is native to hot areas and in Northern Europe it is usually in flower when the Sun is in Leo. The very fact that it is one of the costliest of oils may endear it to the Leo, who will feel that the expense validates his own importance. As we have already seen, it is the supreme oil for Leos to use when a dark cloud passes over their personal Sun, bringing the quality of sunshine with it to help them until they can move out of the darkness.

Virgo

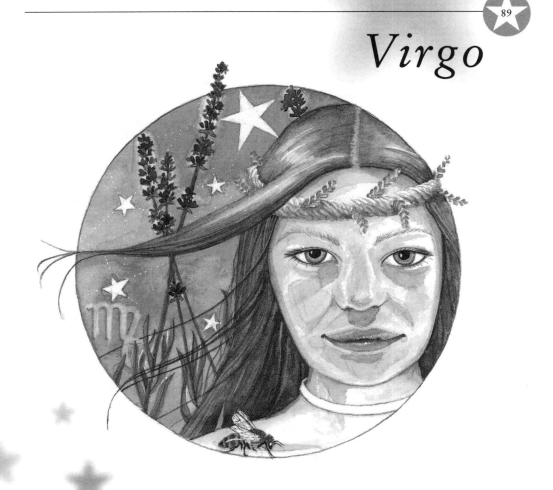

Gathering ripe sheaves at harvest's fullness

She shares her bounty with all Earth's children,

And of herself she gives, unstinting,

Maiden, mother, healer, worker.

Virgo

Virgo Symbol: 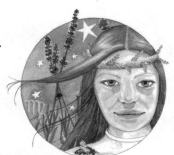 ♍

24th August – 23rd September
Planet: *Mercury/Chiron*
Element: *Earth*
Quality: *Mutable*
Signature Oil: *Lavender*

Virgo is often depicted as a young woman holding a sheaf of wheat, and the various names for this constellation in early civilisations included 'corn seed' as well as 'maiden' or 'young woman'. The Sun moves through this sign during the season of harvest, and Virgo was originally associated with mother-goddesses, suppliers of food and nurture such as the Babylonian earth-goddess, Ninhursaga, and Atargatis, a Syrian fertility goddess and, later in history, the Roman corn-goddess, Demeter (Greek Ceres). The Latin word 'virgo' means a young woman, not necessarily a sexually inexperienced young woman and some of the earliest myths associated with the sign of Virgo concerned earth-goddesses who coupled with the sky-god and gave birth to a world saviour. The story of Isis and Osiris and their son Horus is one such legend, and in Graeco-Roman mythology we find Leto, the mother of Apollo. The existence of such legends made some Romans receptive to the early Christian teachings concerning the Virgin Mary.

Virgo is the sign of service and work and is often described as the sign most concerned with health and healing. This is because ill health was traditionally seen as the converse of work: if you were well, you worked, if you were ill, you could not. We can, of course, make many connections between healing and the idea of service, and you will find many Virgoans in the caring professions, as nurses, care assistants, complementary therapists, house-mothers – wherever people need to be taken care of, you will find Virgos. They have a deep need to feel that they are doing something useful and worthwhile.

Some modern astrologers consider that Chiron, which symbolises the Healer, has strong and obvious connections with Virgo and I agree with this view. Traditionally, however, Mercury is the 'ruling' planet, and I do not think we should wholly discard the old attributions. Both Chironic and Mercurial traits can be seen quite clearly in the Virgoan character.

In this Earth sign, Mercury's influence manifests in a different way to the Air sign, Gemini. The Virgoan keenness of mind shows itself in precision and attention to detail. They tend to be highly organised and make excellent accountants, librarians, indexers or proofreaders, though if taken to extremes this ability can sometimes become nit-picking, critical or even obsessional.

The Virgoan ideal of service often leads these people to put their own needs a poor second to the needs of others and health problems may arise as a result of this. They will work long hours, whether in paid employment or in the service of their family, and carry on even when exhausted. Consequently they can become depleted physically. Anaemia is a common problem and it may be as well to offer advice on foods and nutritional supplements to prevent this. Many Virgoans are chronic worriers and extra liable to stress, while their fascination with everything to do with health and illness makes some into hypochondriacs. Some Virgos will neglect their own creative or intellectual activities if they compete with the interests of their family or others that they are caring for, leading to deep frustrations which they will not openly express. Remember that Chiron is the *Wounded* Healer.

To help them re-establish their strength, you will need to give them some of the nurture that they so unsparingly give to others. (If you are a Virgoan reading this, please try to get on the receiving end of some massage from time to time!)

Physically, Virgo has affinities with the liver, solar plexus and lower digestive tract and these are areas where problems may manifest when the Virgoan overworks or worries excessively. Ulcers and colitis are among the Virgoan problems that can be helped by essential oils, though

I would be inclined to suggest consulting a medical herbalist as well for internal remedies.

Many of the herbs of Mercury, Virgo's planet, are very appropriate: Caraway, Fennel and Peppermint are all helpful for the digestive system, while Lavender will help to induce the relaxation that Virgos so often deny themselves. For the deep nurturing that they may both need and deserve, I would turn to something really luxurious, such as Rose or Jasmine. Sometimes, in their single-minded focus on being of service to others, Virgos tend to deny themselves pleasures and a massage with something really sensuous can remind them that they are as deserving of nurture as anybody else. It also reaffirms their value as a unique and special person, something that Virgos are apt to forget.

★ SIGNATURE OIL

The signature oil is Lavender. This is a herb of Mercury, more specifically, Mercury in his caduceus-carrying role, and everything about it reflects the Virgoan nature: it speaks to us of cleanliness, of linen neatly folded and sweetly scented, of furniture lovingly polished, of children bathed and sweetly put to bed. It is the supremely healing oil – if we could have but a single oil in aromatherapy it would have to be Lavender, for its wide-ranging properties: calming, soothing, antiseptic, antidepressant, wound-healing, to name only a few and in this we can see the influence of Chiron in Virgo, as well as Mercury. For the Virgoan herself, Lavender can ease the tendency to worry, soothe weary muscles after long hours of serving others and promote the restful sleep that this sign needs so much in order to avoid exhaustion in the service of those around them.

Libra

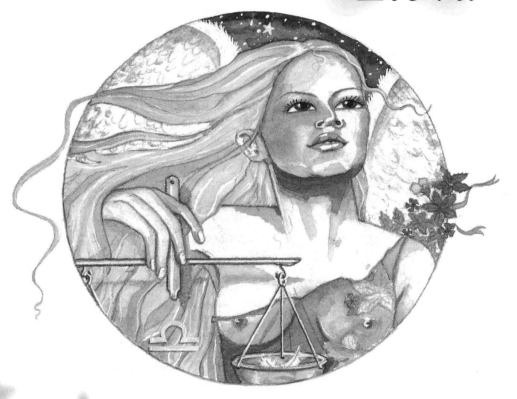

Air-born child of Venus, beauty-loving,

Prizing fairness, seeking balance,

Builder of bridges, loving partner,

Caring, sharing, diplomatic.

Libra

Libra Symbol: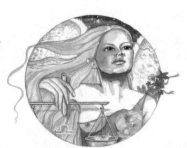
24th September – 23rd October
Planet: *Venus*
Element: *Air*
Quality: *Cardinal*
Signature Oil: *Geranium*

Libra's glyph symbolises a pair of scales and this is the only sign represented by an inanimate object, though many artists down the ages have chosen to place the scales in the hands of a human figure. Early Turkish and Indian manuscripts have a man holding the scales and in mediaeval and Renaissance art allegories of justice showed a woman holding the scales, a tradition perpetuated in the figure crowning the law courts in London. But to earlier civilisations the significance of the scales was even more important than the administration of justice: in Egypt the scales were the attribute of the god Anubis who weighed the heart of a newly deceased person to decide whether they deserved to be admitted to eternal life. The Roman understanding of Libra was that, as the Sun enters this sign at the autumn equinox, Libra held the two halves of the year in balance.

Justice, fairness and balance are, indeed, very important to Librans. They will look at both sides of any argument, try to see the other person's view, try to weigh up every situation and resolve every dispute. Libra is the diplomat and peacekeeper of the Zodiac. A perfect example is the Libran, Mahatma Ghandi, a reformer totally committed to non-violence. The Air quality is very evident here, in the intellectual exercise involved and a certain degree of detachment from the situation to be judged.

But that is far from the whole of Libra, for its planet is Venus, bringing the love of beauty, the arts and creature comforts that we saw in Taurus. Here in this Air sign the influence of Venus is more refined than in earthy Taurus and may show itself as connoisseurship. Librans have impeccable taste – they bring that quality of judgement to bear on their appreciation of beautiful things – but tend towards the informal, both in dress and in organising their home surroundings. A Libran's home will be pleasing to the eye without ever being stuffy.

Libra is first of the 'social' signs, and is associated with the seventh house, the House of Partnership, so it is not surprising that their appreciation of beauty does not stop at beautiful objects – they have an eye for beautiful people, too and are quite often good-looking themselves. Even if not endowed with physical good looks they are among the most charming people you can encounter!

Not surprisingly, Librans excel at partnership, whether it be in romantic/sexual relationships, with friends or business associates, and relate easily with people of all ages – lucky the child that has a Libran father! At its most extreme, their desire to see both sides of a question can lead to indecisiveness and vacillation or putting other people's needs first, to their own detriment (in which they resemble Virgos, though for different reasons).

Many Librans share the Taurean love of good things: food, wine, clothes, etc. but, because the essence of Libra is balance, they are less likely to overindulge. It is when a Libran temporarily loses sight of that sense of balance that health problems tend to arise, due to overwork, overindulgence or mental overload.

Libra is associated with the kidneys and lower back. Needless to say, if there is the slightest suspicion of kidney disease the person should be referred to a medical doctor, though you can use oils to help, too, provided the doctor has no objection. Lower back pain, though, is something that aromatherapy can really help.

When looking for suitable oils to help Librans, it may pay to remember that Venus is the traditional ruler of Libra, as well as Taurus, and to consider many of the oils that were discussed under that sign. (Venus is in fact the only planet that is now generally associated with more than one sign.) So we can look to oils such as Rose, Geranium and

Ylang-Ylang which will appeal to the Libran taste for luxury. For digestive problems, Angelica, Cardamon and Cinnamon are all good digestive aids and Fennel is an excellent detoxifier and diuretic. For low back pain, I would use one of the warming analgesics, such as Marjoram, or Rosemary if the person concerned is overtired and depleted.

It is really important for the Libran to strike up a good rapport with their therapist; in some cases this may prove even more important than the choice of oils.

★ SIGNATURE OIL

The signature oil for Libra is Geranium...or is it? Maybe it is Palmarosa? Truly, only Libra could have *two* signature oils! (Perhaps Gemini could, but Basil seems to suffice.) Geranium suggests itself first, being an oil of Venus, and the supreme balancer in aromatherapy. Its use in perfumery and beauty therapy is typically Venusian, as is its beneficial effect on the female hormone system. However, I have come across a significant proportion of Librans who simply cannot stand the aroma of Geranium, indeed some who are physically allergic to the oil, and in deference to them I offer Palmarosa as an alternative. This is another Venusian oil, and again it is one that is used widely in perfumery, having a delightful and complex aroma somewhere between that of Geranium and Rose. Its uses in beauty therapy are similar to those of Geranium. Librans love to weigh up both sides of a question, to make choices and exercise their discrimination, so if you are a Libran you may enjoy choosing between these oils and deciding which is the special one for you.

Scorpio

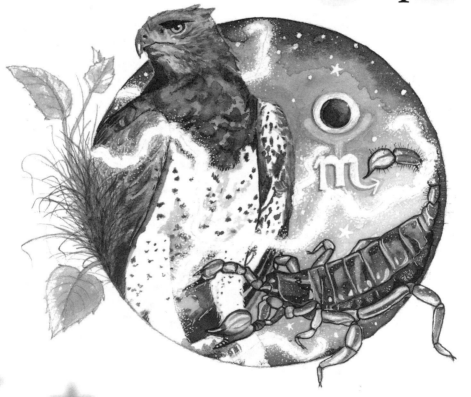

Rising from the deep, the solitary Scorpion
Hugs to his heart his passion's secret.
Leathery shell and lethal tail defend him.
Silence belies the power of love and hate.

Scorpio

Scorpio Symbol: ♏

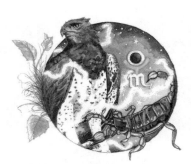

24th October – 22nd November
Planet: *Mars/Pluto*
Element: *Water*
Quality: *Fixed*
Signature Oil: *Patchouli*

Scorpio marks the descent into winter, highlighted by the Celtic festival of Samhain, more generally known as Halloween, and the association with ghosts and ghouls has something in common with Scorpio's nature. The planet that we associate now with the sign is Pluto, representing the underworld, the domain of phantoms, and many of the legends associated with the constellation of Scorpio concern the descent of a hero into some lower world and his eventual return to the light. Modern psychological astrology likens this to the inner journey into the shadow and our emergence with greater self-understanding.

The constellation was called 'Scorpion' or 'The Stinger' by the Sumerians as long as 5,000 years ago and the name has persisted in virtually every tradition. It is fascinating to note that the Mayans, who had no contact with these Middle Eastern civilisations, gave it exactly the same name.

Scorpio often gets a bad press! Maybe because people associate this sign with the 'sting in the tail' but more likely because this is the deepest, most secretive sign in the entire Zodiac. Scorpio people tend to have very strong emotions, but find it difficult to express them and I suspect that this engenders a certain amount of suspicion in many people, to whom they merely appear moody. In this they have much in common with Cancerians, who also hide their vulnerability under a tough shell. They don't make friends easily and prefer to have a small circle of close and trusted friends rather than a wider circle of casual acquaintances.

The same criteria apply to intimate partners: Scorpios will live alone rather than enter a relationship that does not fulfil their need for deep commitment and trust, but once they have made such a decision they will be passionate and faithful. They are often very serious people, quietly determined and with considerable reserves of energy.

The traditional 'ruler' of this sign was Mars, the planet most associated with energy, but whereas in Aries this manifests very openly in physical activity and an adventurous mind, in Scorpio the energy may lay dormant and hidden. Reflecting these differences, the mediaeval astrologers referred to Aries as the 'Day House of Mars' and to Scorpio as Mars' 'Night House'.

Although this is a Water sign, I always feel that there is a smouldering quality in Scorpios, a suggestion of fire underneath. An underwater volcano waiting to erupt would be an apt comparison. Volcanoes are associated with Pluto, Lord of the Underworld, and the majority of astrologers now recognise Pluto as the Planet most closely associated with Scorpio, though as I said in discussing the dual planetary associations in Virgo, we should not forget the older, traditional attributions, for they can still teach us much.

Thinking of the old planetary attribution brings to mind that there is also an alternative to the Scorpion as a symbol for this sign, and that is the Eagle. The Eagle expresses the highest spiritual aspirations of Scorpio, but also the strength, the power and determination that underlies this sign.

Scorpios tend not to ask for help readily. They will self-medicate, or stoically put up with problems until they are no longer tolerable, perhaps through a fear of 'letting go' or losing control, so if you are a practising aromatherapist, you are likely to see Scorpios who are in really urgent need of help. Physically, Scorpio is associated with the urino-genital system, the colon and (in men) the prostate gland, and many people are reluctant to seek early help for problems affecting these areas. When they do, it will often be a matter for the GP or urologist rather than an aromatherapist.

If you use essential oils at home and one of your family or close friends is a Scorpio, you may be able to help them at a much earlier stage. Once you have gained their trust, Scorpios will be more likely to ask you for help. In common with the other two Water signs, they are likely to prefer aromatic baths to massage: not only do these involve their own element, they allow the privacy that Scorpios value so highly.

A depleted Scorpio will benefit from Mars oils, those that bring stimulating warmth, such as Pine, Ginger or Black Pepper. Sun oils might be helpful too: Rosemary is an immediate choice, also Jasmine or Bergamot if there is depression.

★ SIGNATURE OIL

Patchouli parallels the nature of Scorpio in several ways. Firstly, in its depth: it is one of the 'deepest' base-note oils in aromatherapy. Secondly, in its aphrodisiac properties reminding us that Scorpio is a sign profoundly linked to sexuality, both in the Scorpionic nature and the fact that this sign is associated with the genitals. In the South-East Asian countries where Patchouli originates it is traditionally used to treat snake bites and those of poisonous insects...and here we are considering the sign with 'a sting in its tail'!

Sagittarius

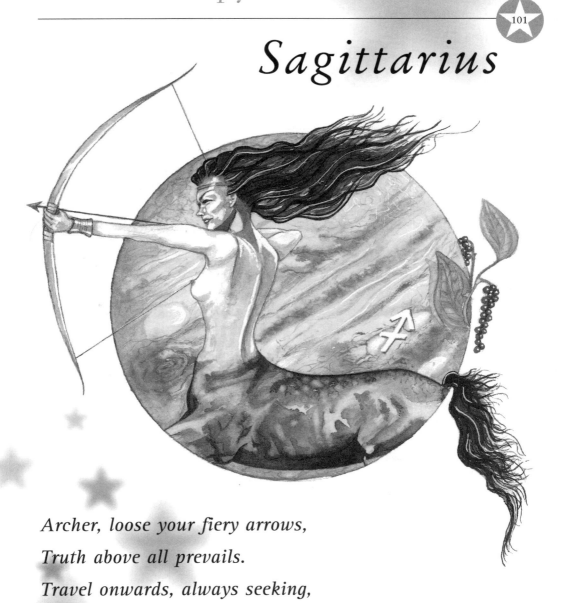

Archer, loose your fiery arrows,

Truth above all prevails.

Travel onwards, always seeking,

Beloved teacher, we honour your great wisdom.

Sagittarius

Sagittarius Symbol: ♐

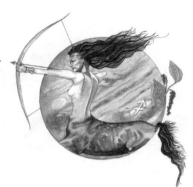

23rd November – 21st December

Planet: *Jupiter*

Element: *Fire*

Quality: *Mutable*

Signature Oil: *Black Pepper*

Sagittarius is the last of the Fire signs, associated less with the Sun than with the fires of mid-winter celebrations. Its time culminates in the winter solstice, and we find festivals involving light – in the form of candles, lanterns or bonfires – all round the world, from Diwali in India to Jewish Hanukkah, the Celtic Yule and the Christian Christmas.

Unlike the majority of constellations forming the Zodiac, there seems to have been little or no consensus on its name. The Greeks called it 'the Archer' as we do today, and the Indians 'the Bow'. Elsewhere it was seen as a horse, though the Chinese identified it as a tiger until fairly recent times when it was renamed Jin Ma or 'Man-Horse' and it is as a Man-Horse, or Centaur, that we recognise Sagittarius today. Some myths identify Sagittarius with Crotus, a satyr whose father was Pan, therefore a two-legged rather than a four-legged being, but Crotus was said to have invented archery, and rode on horseback, so the two may have become merged in the imagination.

In psychological terms, the Centaur represents two sides of human nature: the animal and the divine. We can also understand the Horse part of the Centaur as the traveller, and the Man part as the thinker and, astrologically, this is the sign of the traveller, but also of the teacher and philosopher. In this, Sagittarius has a clear affinity with the planet Jupiter, symbolising expansion, travel, philosophy and religion.

Sagittarians are inquisitive and enthusiastic but, where Aries explores new ground, Sagittarians want to clarify and comprehend. They also want, often passionately, to pass on what they have learned in so doing, and many Sagittarians become teachers. You will find them in the universities where they are most likely to be teaching philosophy, logic or theology and, increasingly, among the spiritual leaders and teachers of esoteric topics. The teacher who travels around the world lecturing, leading workshops, etc., sums up a whole lot of Sagittarian traits in one person!

Truth is something Sagittarians care about deeply, both in their personal dealings and in any writing, speaking or teaching work that they may undertake. In fact, the motivation for such work is often a desire to share what they perceive as truth. But even that may change from time to time as they explore new avenues and discover new philosophies, and they will, indeed, be continually exploring because they want to experience everything.

Outside of their work, they are usually sociable, genuinely interested in other people, open, spontaneous and optimistic. They love conversation, especially if it involves philosophical or metaphysical matters though this can become one-sided: if anybody is willing to listen the Sagittarian will talk at great length about whatever interests them currently. This may sound as if they are overwhelmingly serious, but in fact they have a well-developed sense of humour which may extend to practical jokes and clowning.

In close relationships, too, they value truth almost above anything else. Any suggestion of deceit on the part of a partner is virtually guaranteed to bring the relationship to an end. They tend to look for a partner who is a friend first and foremost, somebody who will share their interests and be prepared to explore and change with them, but their restlessness and love of travel can mitigate against stability. They need a lot of freedom in relationships, and will react strongly against any attempt to limit that freedom. There's also a tendency towards unconventional partnerships, sometimes with a very large difference in age between the people involved – the Sagittarian usually being the elder of the two. This can work well but there is a risk of the relationship becoming a teacher/pupil association rather than a meeting of equals.

Sagittarians are most often very physical people, energetic, quick-moving, strong. This sign is associated with the hips and thighs – with their connotations of travel, running, forward motion. But strains or injuries to the thigh are unlikely to be the main reason for a Sagittarian to look for help from an aromatherapist. Sciatica is a problem where massage and baths with essential oils could be very helpful, but Sagittarians are more likely to be needing help with exhaustion, even burn-out because they will push themselves to the limit and beyond in pursuit of their various enthusiasms. Jet lag is a frequent hazard for the modern, globe-trotting Sagittarius. Jupiter oils such as Marjoram and Nutmeg have a comforting warmth but if a Sagittarian is really depleted, Mars oils such as Ginger, Pine or Black Pepper (the Sagittarian signature oil) will be more helpful. Occasionally, you may need to select calming oils, when their passion excites them to the point where they are jittery and insomniac: Rosewood would be a beautiful choice here, because of its association with Jupiter and the higher mind.

★ SIGNATURE OIL

Black Pepper reflects the ardent nature of Sagittarius. Tonic, stimulant, fiery, the aroma has a directness that reminds us of the Sagittarian single-mindedness and love of truth. This is an oil that 'gets straight to the point' like the Archer's arrow, whether the 'point' is a stiff, painful muscle or a tired mind. It is particularly appropriate to the athletic Sagittarian and is often used in massage blends both before and after training or performance to warm and tonify the muscles. For the travel-loving Sagittarian, Black Pepper combats fatigue and jet lag and helps them to continue their journey with renewed vigour.

Capricorn

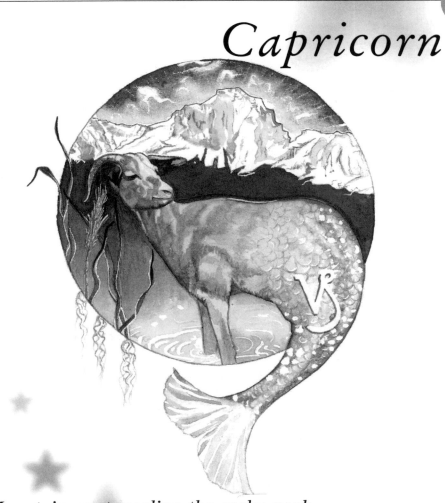

Mountain-goat, scaling the rocky peak,

Step by slow step from Earth's greatest depths,

Leap suddenly to reach your lofty goal,

Wise man, old man, forever young man.

Capricorn

Capricorn Symbol: ♑
22nd December – 20th January
Planet: *Saturn*
Element: *Earth*
Quality: *Cardinal*
Signature Oil: *Vetivert*

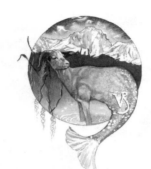

Capricorn, the Goat, is the deepest of the Earth signs. The mythical creature for which the sign is named, is no ordinary goat, but a sea-goat, with a goat's front half and the hindquarters of a fish, symbolically representing Capricorn's ability to both plumb the depths and rise to the heights. The Babylonians first named the constellation 'goat-fish', the Indians 'sea-monster' while the Greeks called it 'goat-horned' and identified it with Pan, half goat and half man, but when threatened by a monster, Typhon, Pan hid in a river and turned his lower half into a fish.

The goat strives to get to the top of the mountain, whatever that may mean for each individual. While some Capricorns may be very ambitious and career-orientated, others may transcend worldly ambition and we find many poets, philosophers and spiritual teachers in this sign. "Feet in the earth and head in the clouds" is often a good description of the Capricornian but never forget that the goat can leap. These people will climb painstakingly from one objective to the next if needs be to achieve their goal, but they may also make huge and unpredictable bounds.

The planet with which Capricorn has special affinity is Saturn which represents time, responsibilities, boundaries, authority, etc., and Saturn people tend to value tradition and like order, both in their physical surroundings and in work, friendships and relationships. They take very seriously any responsibility which they take on, whether that is in connection with their work, or as a parent, friend or mentor. Capricorn people often show immense courage in defending others, if they perceive a threat to their family, friends, social group or ideal they believe in. Paradoxically, most

Capricorns have a crazy sense of humour – the giddy side of the goat.

The part of the body associated with Capricorn is the knees, but it is as well to bear in mind the whole bone structure when working with these people. Remember that Capricorn's affinity-planet is Saturn which symbolises everything to do with structure. You may well find Capricorns suffering from pain in or around the knee joint: be meticulous in determining whether this is due to problems affecting the muscles or tendons around the knee or the knee joint itself. If you are in any doubt (particularly if you are not a trained therapist) leave well alone until the cause has been ascertained by an osteopath, chiropractor or other suitably trained practitioner. Once you are assured that you can do no harm, try massaging around the knee with warming oils – perhaps Sun, Jupiter or even Mars ones. It will often be advisable to refer Capricorn people to an osteopath or chiropractor for other reasons: as aromatherapists we are not equipped to help with problems affecting the skeletal structure. We may help, by massaging the areas around an affected joint, but actual manipulation needs to be carried out by somebody with an appropriate training.

Saturn is also connected with the skin (because it forms the outer boundary of the body) and this is, of course, an area where aromatherapy is highly effective and totally appropriate.

We should bear in mind also the influence of Saturn on the mental and emotional well-being of Capricorns: their sense of responsibility can lead them to stay in relationships that have long ceased to be meaningful, whether for the sake of apparent stability or because they genuinely believe that this is in the interests of their children. Conversely, the Pan-like part of Capricorn sometimes manifests as conducting affairs while maintaining a sterile marriage. Then again, remembering the goat and its propensity for sudden leaps, the Capricorn may abandon a partner suddenly and without warning. Any of these situations can lead to great stress – both for the Capricorn and for everyone else involved.

Another manifestation of the Saturn influence is taking on too much and leaving themselves depleted. They need to feel useful and leave themselves open to being exploited by people who will take advantage of that need. Capricorns will often take on positions of authority, teaching for example, or managerial positions in business or industry where they will work themselves to a standstill rather than leave a task unfinished. They are punctilious in their attention to detail and can worry over small discrepancies to a degree that is out of all proportion to the situation.

They may also be quite restrained emotionally, reluctant to show their feelings or to talk about themselves. Many of Capricorn's health problems have their origin in stress but they may be resistant to discussing this and you will need to be extremely patient and tactful if you are to help them effectively. They tend to ignore physical problems and carry on stoically, or have a somewhat spartan attitude, so they need encouragement to pamper themselves.

Helpful oils are likely to be Sun or Jupiter ones, even Mars oils to warm and tonify weak or painful joints. Birch, which is one of the few oils attributed to Saturn, is analgesic and anti-inflammatory, so it would be another good choice for joint pain. The goat or Pan side of Capricorn does appreciate the physical comfort of massage and, once they have convinced themselves that aromatherapy is actually of benefit to them, they are likely to return regularly for treatment. They will almost certainly appreciate oils with a deep aroma, such as Cedarwood or the signature oil, Vetivert.

★ SIGNATURE OIL

Vetivert reflects perfectly the earthy nature of Capricorn, even to the extent that it is extracted from the roots of the parent plant. It is dark brown in colour, thick and viscous in texture and the aroma is dark, earthy, smoky and in some ways almost more animal-like than you would expect from a plant – an echo, perhaps of the Goat-like nature of this sign. It is valuable for rheumatic and arthritic pain, reminding us that joint pains are common among Capricorns, and it is also used in skincare, often in masculine toiletries. In the Far East, where the fragrant grass that gives us this oil is grown, it is known as the 'Oil of Tranquillity' and may help the conscientious Capricorn who worries unduly about work or personal issues.

Aquarius

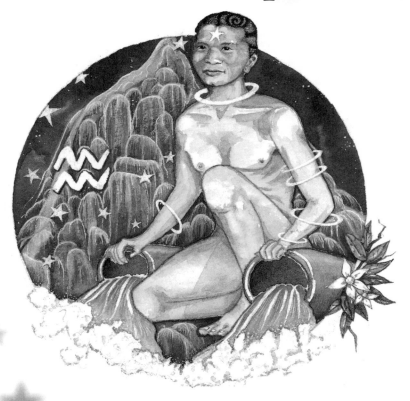

Airborne carrier of water,

Bring us the new, eternally surprise us.

Ignite our hopes, our wildest notions.

Dream-friend, guide us to our future.

Aquarius

Aquarius Symbol: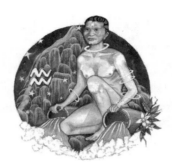
21st January – 19th February
Planet: *Uranus*
Element: *Air*
Quality: *Fixed*
Signature Oil: *Neroli*

Aquarius is the last of the Air signs, which is possibly confusing as its name means 'Water Bearer'. Perhaps it would be helpful to think of airy clouds carrying rain. The Babylonians named the constellation 'the Giant' but associated it with Ea, one of their four creator-gods, and the Sumerians before them identified it with Enki, who poured the waters of life over the Earth. The Greeks called it 'water pot' and various civilisations have called it by similar names since.

Present-day astrologers associate Aquarius with Uranus, the planet of the unconventional, the unexpected, even of revolution, first discovered in 1781. Although the glyph for Aquarius is intended to represent the water flowing from the water bearer's pot, it can also be read as a flash of lightning, representing the revolutionary nature of the sign. People born under this sign often appear eccentric or non conformist, but they may well be geniuses! The 'absent-minded professor' – intellectually brilliant but totally unable to cope with the day-to-day practicalities of life – is an Aquarian archetype.

Aquarians are attracted to new ideas, new technologies, anything unusual or unorthodox and are often ahead of their times: they may well be mocked for their 'lunatic fringe' enthusiasm for some new form of healing or theory of physics, only to find their ideas accepted as mainstream a decade or so later. They tend to dislike routine and will be much happier working in an unconventional setting that offers plenty of variety or being self-employed.

Many Aquarians are social reformers though their revolutionary ideas tend to stay that way – as ideas. They are less likely to be found storming the barricades than writing a treatise on housing, disability or mental health. Sometimes, though, the Aquarian suspicion of the status quo manifests as a negative, disgruntled, anti-establishment attitude. They may be aggressively nonconformist, drop-outs or social misfits. As we have seen before, the potential of any sign can manifest in both positive and negative ways and this is, perhaps, more obvious in Aquarius than some of the other signs. However, most Aquarians, as you might expect, are somewhere between these extremes.

They have a certain reputation for coldness and aloofness which may be because they are reluctant to confide their thoughts or feelings to anybody but their very closest friends, who are probably few in number. Otherwise, friendships tend to be sociable rather than intimate and are often based on shared interests – maybe humanitarian or political. They do tend to be very independent people, setting great store by their privacy and are often quite happy to live alone, sometimes genuinely reclusive. Those who are not are usually rather easy-going and often have a quirky sense of humour.

In relationships, the Aquarian can be equally unpredictable and nonconformist, sometimes tending to sexual ambiguity. They tend not to rush into marriage or relationships, being quite self-sufficient, but when they do will often choose surprising partners. Mental rapport is often a more important consideration in such a choice than any other factor. Ideally, they need a partner who will respect their independence and the need to be alone at times.

Physically, Aquarius is connected with the lower legs, particularly the ankles and the circulation in this part of the body, so look out for problems in this area. Varicose veins are a common problem, and strains of the Achilles tendon, sprained ankles or ankles swollen due to fatigue and standing for long periods of time are also likely. Though in my experience Aquarians are less likely to look to aromatherapy for help with health or other problems than many of the other signs. Aquarians are also more susceptible than some of the other signs to nervous disorders and for some of them it may be that counselling or psychotherapy is a more appropriate form of help than aromatherapy. The sheer physicality of massage is unlikely to appeal to them and they are more likely to be attracted to the cerebral nature of homoeopathy or, conversely, to the latest and most way-out healing system to hit the alternative scene!

If, however, you find yourself offering help to an Aquarian you might try to engage their interest by telling them about the chemistry of essential oils, the process of distillation or the theories of blending, which will arouse their curiosity. Deep, grounding oils, particularly those associated with Saturn, can help these rather 'floaty' people to connect with their physical bodies.

Vetivert would be a very good choice, also Cypress which is a good circulatory tonic and recommended for varicose veins. To tone the ankles or strengthen them when recovering from a sprain, massage or hot compresses with warming Sun or Mars oils would be good, though these should not be used in the immediate aftermath of a sprain: at that stage, cold compresses of Camomile are the best treatment.

★ SIGNATURE OIL

The ethereal nature of Neroli reflects the very best of the Aquarian character. Neroli is both a meditation aid and an aphrodisiac, as well as being one of the most subtle and exquisite perfumes. To many Aquarians, the meditative quality of the oil will have an immediate appeal, but it is important for these mentally orientated people to remember their bodies and treat them kindly, and the more Venusian qualities of Neroli can help them do so. It is a wonderful oil for insomnia, a problem which afflicts many Aquarians. Finally, although the signature oil for any sign is not necessarily the 'favourite' oil of people born under that sign, in the case of Neroli it seems to be universally beloved of Aquarians.

Pisces

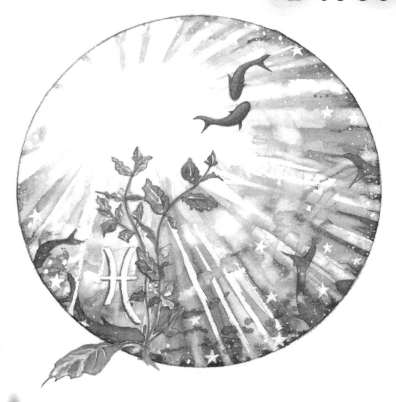

End of journey, new beginning,
The Fishes pull in opposite directions,
Dissolving, dying, melting, merging,
Becoming one with Neptune's ocean.

Pisces

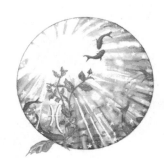

Pisces Symbol: ♓
20th February – 20th March
Planet: *Neptune*
Element: *Water*
Quality: *Mutable*
Signature Oil: *Melissa*

Pisces, the Fishes, is the last of the Water signs. Its quality, Mutable, tells us that, of the three, Pisces is the one which is most ready to change and this is perhaps of greater significance in Pisces than in the other Mutable signs. For in Pisces we reach the end of the annual cycle of the Zodiac. At the end of Pisces we do not merely move into a new element and a new sign, but into a new astrological year and into the fiery, 'beginning' sign of Aries. Pisces can be likened to the primordial ocean in which all is dissolved in order to facilitate the creation of something new.

Piscean people reflect something of this in their fluid natures. Elusive, deeply emotional, sometimes moody, one astrologer-friend describes Pisces as 'the weepiest sign of the Zodiac'. Often highly intuitive, empathetic and compassionate, they feel other people's sufferings as keenly as their own and can in some instances be self-sacrificing. Indeed, one of the difficulties of Pisces is an inability to establish boundaries – there are times when it is hard for a Piscean to know where 'I' ends and 'the Other' begins. Some have a tendency to live their lives through other people.

The glyph for Pisces represents two fish swimming in opposite directions, and Pisceans are notoriously difficult to 'pin down'. They can find it difficult to arrive at decisions, swinging first this way and then that, as if being carried by the tide first in one direction and then in the other.

On the credit side, Neptune, the planet associated with Pisces, can deeply inspire great idealism, spiritual aspirations or artistic inspiration, but the negative of this is that Pisceans can be self-deluding or duplicitous.

In personal relationships, Pisceans are idealistic, intensely romantic and will probably be very sensitive to their partner's feelings but may not always be realistic in their choice of partner and suffer intensely when things go wrong. Problems may flare up because Pisceans are not very good at explaining things and – because they are themselves so intuitive and empathetic – tend to think that other people know what they are thinking without being told. The ideal relationship for a Piscean is with a partner who is stable enough to cope with their changeability and this is a considerable challenge as they tend to change their minds, alter arrangements and swing from one extreme of mood to another with perplexing speed. They often need solitude and privacy, and can seem very detached at times.

Pisceans are natural actors – their empathetic nature makes it easy for them to get inside any character they are asked to play, and we also find many Pisceans in the other arts, as painters, poets and musicians. But it is as dancers that they most characteristically embody their sign...think of the fluidity of water and the grace of a dancer like the Piscean, Rudolf Nureyev, and it will not surprise you that this sign is associated with the feet.

This may express itself as a gift, or conversely as a weakness. If a Piscean seeks your help with aromatherapy, you may find that they have pain or damage to the feet, or a foot infection such as athlete's foot or verrucas. They will respond very positively to reflexology, which many aromatherapists use as an adjunct to massage with essential oils. Pisces is also related to the lymphatic system and fluid retention can be a problem. Lymph drainage massage with essential oils of Rosemary and Geranium in equal proportions is very effective here, with Birch or Celery as alternative choices.

Pisces people are more likely, though, to be looking for help with problems of emotional origin and, being influenced by Neptune, addiction of one kind or another is often involved, even if it is only to chocolate! Addiction may not always be to a physical substance, but could equally be to an idea or to obsessive fantasies.

Pisceans will enjoy massage more as an expression of your caring than for the physical comfort. Their natural element being water, aromatic baths are the absolute ideal therapy for them, so think about making up bath blends that they can use at home. Depending on the nature of their problems, Sun or Jupiter oils will often be very helpful: a Piscean in trouble frequently needs the psychological warmth that these can bring. Bergamot, Jasmine and Frankincense come to mind, as does Melissa, which is the signature oil of Pisces.

★ SIGNATURE OIL

Pisces is perhaps the most archetypal of the Water signs, and Melissa is the most 'watery' of essential oils. The plant itself has such a high water content that the extraction of oil from it requires vast quantities of plant material to obtain a little oil, hence its high cost. The healing and comforting properties reflect the compassionate nature of the Piscean but Pisceans themselves are more than usually susceptible to depression, and at such times they need comforting and healing themselves. As an antidepressant Melissa reigns supreme. Gerard wrote that, "It maketh the heart merry and joyful and strengtheneth the vitall spirit," and a Swiss manuscript by an unknown author says that it "chases away black thoughts".

Astrological
Aromatherapy

The sky gods

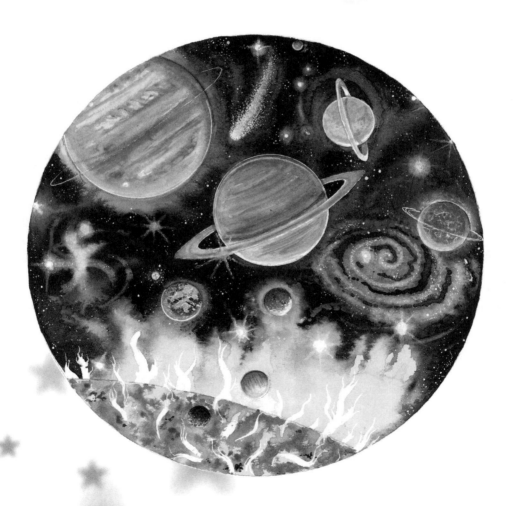

The sky gods

Starting nearest the Sun and working outwards the planets are: Mercury, Venus, (Earth), Mars, Jupiter, Saturn, Uranus, Neptune and Pluto. The Sun and Moon, known in astrology as the 'Lights' are not planets, of course, scientifically speaking, but are treated as if they were planets in interpreting a chart, and are the two most important.

The names of all the planets are those of Graeco-Roman gods and goddesses and the myths surrounding those gods give us clues as to what they symbolise in a chart. For example, Mercury was the messenger of the gods and the position of Mercury in a chart tells us something about a person's powers of communication, while Venus in the chart tells us about their attitude to love, beauty, creature comforts and the arts.

When we look at the planets in somebody's natal chart, they are not all equal in their influence: the Sun and Moon take pride of place, followed by the 'personal planets', Mercury, Venus and Mars. The sign in which a planet is placed also influences the way that planet works in the chart. Each of the planets is associated with a sign which has something in common with that planet in terms of character/archetype. When we see a planet in the sign it is linked with, the influence of that planet will be strong because the nature of the sign and that of the planet are in harmony. Conversely, if it is in the opposite sign, its influence will be weaker. For each planet, there is also another pair of signs in which it will manifest less or more strongly, dependent on the nature of the sign, but these are seldom used in modern astrology.

To understand this, it may be helpful to think of the planets as actors in the play of life and the signs as the environment in which they can play their role: if, for example, a fiery planet such as Mars is placed in a Fire sign, it can function most effectively, while in a Water sign it risks having its energy extinguished; in an Air sign it might be blown away, and in an Earth sign it has to work rather harder than in its own element. Conversely, a watery planet such as the Moon or Neptune is not favourably placed in a Fire sign, etc. I am sure you can work out the logic of these associations for yourself.

Traditionally, the planet associated with a sign was described as the 'Ruler' of the sign, because astrology as we know it today developed long ago in civilisations with a hierarchical structure, and the early astrologers imagined that the Universe was organised in the same way. The gods were very real to them and very powerful. They could easily imagine those gods literally controlling the great celestial creatures.

Our view of astrology today is more symbolic, more metaphysical. We see the great gods of Olympus as archetypes of character. I like the term 'planetary *affinity*', coined by Jeff Mayo, as opposed to Rulership but 'Ruler' remains the usual term in astrological texts, so I mention it here to avoid confusion.

However, the names of the planets, corresponding to those of the gods of Olympus, are revealing and are important in understanding what each planet symbolises because we can look at the myths concerning each of these gods in terms of archetypes of character. This way of looking at astrology, which owes much to the work of Carl Jung, has been further developed by psychologist/astrologers such as Liz Greene and Howard Sasportas, among others, and is obviously more valuable to us in allying astrology and aromatherapy than the deterministic beliefs of earlier times.

The Sun

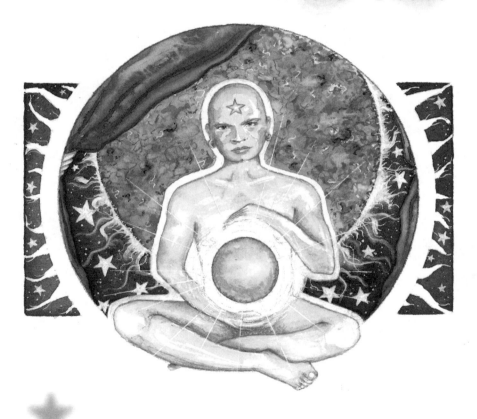

Great Sol, centre of our universe,
Bringer of light and warmth and joy,
Help us to find our own true centre
As we journey to the greater Light.

The Sun ☉

Our Sun is a star, the one around which our Solar system has evolved. As stars go it is not very big but, if we compare it to the size of the Earth, its volume is 330,000 times that of our home planet. Astronomers calculate that the temperature at the Sun's surface is 5800°C while in the centre this rises to 15 million degrees. Here on Earth we are some 93 million miles from the Sun, far enough away to experience its incredible heat as comfortable warmth.

To early civilisations the Sun was a god, and by far the most important and powerful one: Shamash to the Babylonians, Amun-Ra to the Egyptians, Mithras to the Persians and Tonatiuh to the Aztecs. The disappearance of the god each night and his reappearance each morning gave rise to the myths of death and resurrection which stand at the heart of so many religions. To most of these peoples the Sun was male, often the consort of the female Moon, though to some Native American tribes and Australian aboriginal people, the Sun was a powerful goddess. In Japan, too, the Sun is a goddess and the Moon is male.

To the Greeks, the Sun was Helios and to the Romans Apollo though, strangely, neither of these was a supreme god, being less important than Zeus/Jupiter.

The preeminence that earlier people gave to these deities recognised the fact that the Sun is central to life on Earth. Without it, life as we know it could not exist on this planet. There would be perpetual darkness and temperatures so cold we can hardly imagine them, ⁻270°C, but the Sun provides us with the light and warmth which are necessary for all forms of life, from the simplest cells to the most complex mammals (and that includes us!).

Plants depend on sunlight to create the raw materials they need in order to live and grow and reproduce themselves. Imagine a plant that has been kept out of the light and it will demonstrate this dramatically: it quickly turns yellow and then white, because without light it cannot make green chlorophyll cells, and if it is not quickly brought back into the light, it will die because it cannot make any of the other basic materials of plant life.

A plant is a miniature chemical factory which takes oxygen, nitrogen and other materials from the air around it and the soil in which it is growing and converts them into the compounds it needs for its life processes, using energy from sunlight to do so. This process is called photosynthesis, from the Greek *photo* meaning light, and *synthesis* meaning to put together. More complex lifeforms can't do this, so they depend on plants for their food. This is true whether they eat the plants directly, or eat other creatures that feed on plants, or both.

As this book is about aromatherapy as well as celestial bodies, it is worth remembering that essential oils are products of photosynthesis too. The oils are made by plants to repel predators, to attract pollinating insects, to combat disease and for other purposes that we are far from understanding. If you consider the chemical complexity of essential oils – Rose, for example, contains more than 300 chemical compounds – you can begin to comprehend the awesome nature of photosynthesis.

And none of this would be possible without the Sun.

The Sun is central to astrology, too.

Ancient astronomers/astrologers thought it was a hot, dry planet and placed it in natal charts accordingly; even so, they acknowledged its central role by regarding it as the most important feature of the chart. The Sun and Moon are often referred to in astrology as the 'Lights' to distinguish them from the planets.

The Sun in a person's birth chart represents their true self, the core of their being, just as the physical Sun is the radiant core of the solar system. Other factors in the chart will modify this, particularly the position of the Ascendant and the Moon, which we will look at elsewhere, but that part of ourselves which is represented by the Sun is our essence. In infancy, our character is often closer to that suggested by the Moon in our natal chart, but as we mature we ideally become more like our Sun, a journey which can be compared to what Carl Jung named the process of individuation, or becoming our true selves.

The Sun is particularly associated with the sign of Leo and is powerful in a chart when it is in this sign, also in Aries. Conversely it is weaker in the opposite sign of Aquarius and in Libra.

Plants which are associated with the Sun include Angelica, Benzoin, Bergamot, Calendula, Cinnamon, Frankincense, Grapefruit, Helichrysum, Jasmine, Mandarin, Myrrh, Orange, Rosemary and St John's Wort – not an essential oil but a really valuable infused oil.

You may well find some of the above oils appropriate in helping people born in Leo, though of course they will be valuable for natives of any of the signs, depending on their needs at any given moment. Depression is not at all uncommon among Leo people. When they feel that "the Sun has gone out of my life" it can be very difficult for them to recover from the black mood that engulfs them, and Jasmine is one of the best oils to gently restore their confidence.

The Moon

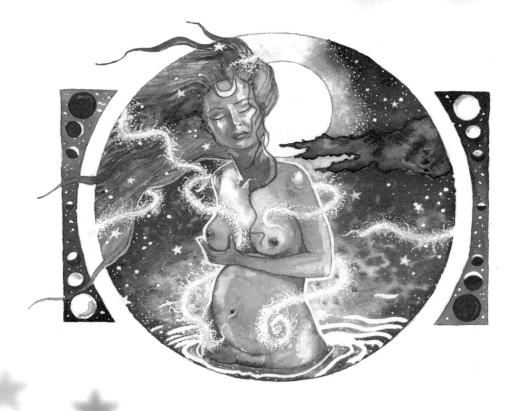

Silver lady, maiden and mother,

Consort of Sol, queen of the waters,

Bring us deep dreams, bless our imagination.

Nurture our hearts and heal our deepest yearning.

The Moon ☽

The Moon is our nearest neighbour in space at 238,000 miles away from the Earth, something highlighted by the fact that it is the only object in the sky on which humans have, so far, trodden. The Moon was long thought to have once been part of Earth, but analysis of rocks brought back by lunar probes suggest that this is not so, and that it was formed in space nearby and at some point pulled into an orbit around Earth.

Earth's only satellite, it travels around us in just over 27 days though, as the Earth is travelling round the Sun at the same time, 29 days elapse between one Full Moon and the next. The regularity of the Moon's phases made it a useful way of measuring time in spans longer than the 24-hour pattern marked by the Sun, especially to agricultural people. Animal bones with the Moon's phases notched on them have been dated to as far back as 35000 BC, and most of the earliest known calendars were lunar, dividing the year into 13 months of about 28 days. More complex calendars combined both solar and lunar elements, but it is quite easy to find lunar calendars nowadays.

Just as the Sun in mythology is most often personified as a male figure, we find the Moon almost always portrayed as female: the consort of the Sun, a mother, or sometimes grandmother, but also in many myths an untouchable virgin. This perception of the Moon as female is undoubtedly linked to its cycle of waxing and waning: long, long ago people observed that the time from one Full Moon to the next corresponded very closely to women's menstrual cycles. They saw the Moon grow large, as in pregnancy, and shrink again to maidenly slenderness at the New Moon and found parallels in both human and animal life. They observed the influence of the Moon on tides and rainfall, which was vital to the survival of their crops, their livestock and themselves, and so the Moon became a goddess, a protector of women, a symbol of fertility.

Thus, in astrology, the Moon came to represent the feminine and particularly the Mother. In modern astrology we see the Moon as symbolising our feminine self and the unconscious, the realms of emotion, feeling and desires as well as the Mother – our biological mother, our experience of receiving nurture as a child and of giving nurture as an adult. This is true of both men and women, for we all embody both masculine and feminine in our character.

The position of the Moon in a birth chart is marked in exactly the same way as those of the planets and the Sun and can tell us a great deal about how a person will react emotionally. This can be extremely helpful in aromatherapy if we are trying to help with emotional difficulties, or physical problems that have their origin in emotional issues (even though the person looking for help may not realise, or may not acknowledge that this is where the root of their problems lies).

Our sense of security is very much linked to the Moon's sign, too: for example, people with the Moon in an Air sign will feel comforted by talking about their problems, while those with Moon in an Earth sign are more comforted by touch. Knowing this can help us with the management of aromatherapy treatments when we can understand why one person may want to talk for some time before feeling ready for a massage or may want to talk throughout the treatment, while another can hardly wait to get onto the massage table and is completely at ease with a companionable silence.

Because the Moon moves so quickly through the signs, it is a little harder to establish an individual's Moon sign than it is to find out their Sun sign: you will need to know the time and place of their birth as well as the date, but once you know these two facts an ephemeris for the year of their birth will quickly show you where the Moon was, astrologically speaking, when they were born. Of course, suitable computer software will do this, too.

The Moon moves through all 12 of the signs of the Zodiac between one New Moon and the next, passing through each sign in a little over two days, and this can be helpful in determining the timing of certain treatments. The Moon's position may not always make a great deal of difference to your choice of oils or the type of treatment offered but it is worth bearing in mind that the areas of the body associated with each sign of the Zodiac tend to be at their most vulnerable when the Moon is passing through that sign. As long ago as the fourth century BC Hippocrates taught that a physician should never operate on a part of the body governed by the sign that the Moon was in at the time. Although surgical operations are far from our remit as aromatherapists we might consider arranging treatment in the days just before the Moon moves into a sign to strengthen the relevant parts of the body as a form of prevention.

The phase of the Moon is important for some kinds of treatments too: massage and oil intended to decongest or detoxify will be far more effective when the Moon is waning (i.e. after Full Moon and before the next New Moon) as will treatment for warts, veruccas and fungal infections of the skin. Conversely, treatments to tonify and strengthen the body, after an accident or illness for example, are more effective when the Moon is waxing, between New Moon and Full Moon. These principles were applied in England as long ago as the eighth century. The same principles apply in skincare: face-packs, masks and other treatments intended to decongest and cleanse are most effective when the Moon is waning; while toning, firming or moisturising work is more effective when it is waxing. However, *all* kinds of skin treatment are beneficial when the Moon is in Capricorn.

Obviously, it isn't always possible to arrange aromatherapy on the most appropriate dates, but perhaps if you have not been getting the results you hoped for from a particular course of treatment it would be well worth considering. A lunar calendar or an ephemeris will show you which sign the Moon is in at any given time and when it moves into the following sign and you can arrange your treatment sessions accordingly.

The Moon is strong in the signs of Cancer and Taurus and weak in the opposite signs of Capricorn and Scorpio.

Plants that are associated with the Moon are classified by herbalists as 'cold and moist'. Many of them are not plants that we use in aromatherapy, but those that we do include Melissa, Lemon, Lime and the various varieties of Camomile. These are among the most soothing of all essential oils and Camomile, in particular, is one of the safest and most appropriate oils for treating children, in complete accordance with the Moon's symbolic role of mother.

Mercury

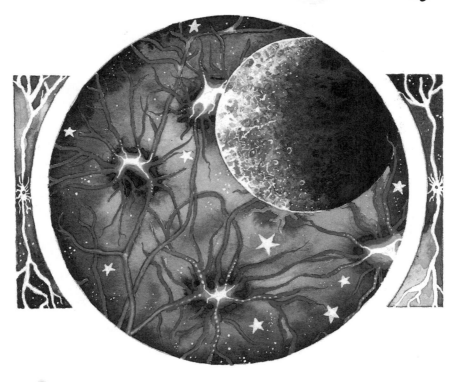

Wing-heeled messenger, artful trickster,

Guide of souls and subtle healer,

Ever-changing, never resting,

Grant us keen minds and crystal speech.

Mercury ☿

Mercury is the nearest planet to the Sun, averaging about 36 million miles from our star. It is the smallest of the 'traditional' planets (i.e. those that can be seen without a telescope) with a diameter of about 3,000 miles. It takes a little over three months to complete its elliptical orbit round the Sun, so seen from Earth it appears to be travelling through the sky faster than any of the other planets, though it is not always easy to see in the sky due to its small size and closeness to the Sun. It is most easily sighted in the evening in spring time, or in the early morning in autumn.

This appearance of speed led it to be associated with the idea of a messenger, particularly the Messenger of the Gods – we always want our messages delivered quickly and the ancient gods were presumed to feel the same. The early Sumerians called the planet Gud, the Babylonians called it Shut and made it sacred to Nab, the God of Scribes and the Egyptians identified it with Thoth. The Greeks called it Hermes, the Romans Mercurius, and between them gave us the classical image of Mercury with wings on his ankles, and the mythology surrounding the Messenger of the Gods.

He was imagined as eternally young – a 'Boy God' – perhaps because of the small size of the planet, perhaps because in maturing he might have lost the youthful attribute of speed or grown tired of running errands for the more senior gods! This idea of the messenger as a youth has persisted down the ages: think of Ariel in Shakespeare's *Tempest*, the errand boy in Victorian times...or the motor-cycle courier today.

So, in astrology, Mercury has come to symbolise intelligence, our ability to understand and communicate, whether in speech, writing or any other way, also communications in the sense of travel, postal systems, telephones, etc.

The position of Mercury in a birth chart tells us about the individual's mental approach, their ability to learn and to communicate and their manner of doing so. As a Boy God, Mercury is particularly associated with our formative years, when we learn first to speak, then to read and write.

The Winged Messenger was also a prankster – a clever one – a thief and a liar from earliest infancy, in many ways resembling the cunning trickster Coyote in Native American mythology. The legends tell us that on the very day he was born he stole his brother Apollo's herd of cattle and drove them backwards into a cave, so that their footprints looked as if they were coming out. When Apollo discovered his loss and accused Mercury, he said, "What, *me*? But I'm only a baby. I can't even climb out of my cradle!"

The trickster side of Mercury can perhaps best be observed at the times when the planet is Retrograde: in other words, when it appears to be moving backwards (like Apollo's cattle!). Of course, the planet is not really moving backwards, this is an optical illusion involving the way we see the planet against the background of other stars while Earth itself is also moving through space, but the effects are as tangible as if it were literal fact. Mercury is seen to be Retrograde three or four times each year, for approximately three weeks each time, and at these times communication of all kinds is often disrupted: trains may run late, packages go astray in the mail, computers malfunction, and messages are misunderstood. During Mercury Retrogrades we need to take extra care that everything we say or write is clearly expressed and fully understood. It is wise to avoid signing any legal documents or entering into any binding contracts at these times.

Where Mercury was Retrograde at the time of a person's birth you will often find that person had difficulty learning to read or write, is dyslexic, was late learning to talk or has a speech impediment of some kind.

Mercury has a special affinity with the sign of Gemini, which is also associated with eloquence, wit and verbal fluency and is considered strong in that sign, and in Virgo, and weak in the opposite signs of Sagittarius and Pisces. As well as Gemini, it has an affinity with Virgo, for there is another side to Mercury's character.

Mercury not only carried messages between the gods of Olympus, he was the only god who could move freely between Earth and the

Underworld (Hades) and so became the *psychopompos* – the guide who conducted souls between the two realms. In this role he is parallel to the Egyptian, Anubis, and both are depicted carrying the caduceus – two serpents twined round a rod, which symbolised the coming together of opposites. We know the caduceus today as the symbol of healing, medicine and doctors. Perhaps this came about because Mercury was able to lead souls up out of Hades, as well as attending them at the time of death. The sign Virgo is also associated with health and healing, so there is a natural link between the planet and the sign. It is interesting to note here that mediaeval astrologers believed the guardian angel of Mercury was the Archangel Raphael, the Healer, not Gabriel who was both messenger and psychopomp in the Judeo-Christian tradition.

Mercury is traditionally associated with the nervous system, the means by which the brain and body communicate with each other.

It has an affinity with plants that are mentally stimulating, and those that have something mercurial about their habit of growth. They include Basil, Caraway, Celery, Clary, Fennel, Lavender, Myrtle, Parsley, Peppermint and Thyme.

Astrological Aromatherapy

Venus

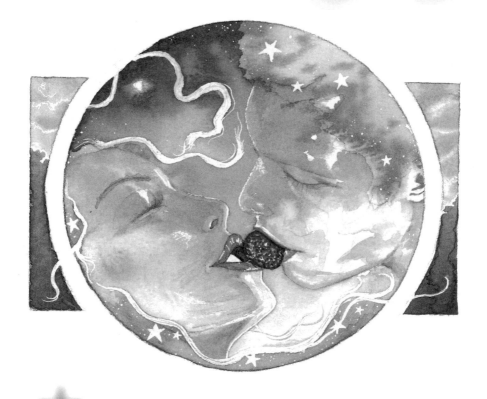

Sea-born goddess, beauty incarnate,

Lover of beauty, lover of love itself,

Delight us with touch and taste and perfume,

Music's airs and love's sweet sharing.

Venus ♀

Travelling outwards from the centre of our solar system, the next planet we come to is Venus, about 67 million miles from the Sun. Venus is far larger than Mercury but smaller than Earth and takes approximately nine months to travel round the Sun. Its appearance is of a very beautiful, bright star, easy to see in the sky and sometimes known as the 'Evening Star' because it is often the first to become visible after dusk. It is also, though, often the first star visible in the morning, and because of this the ancient astronomers sometimes thought it was two stars and often gave feminine attributes to its evening manifestation and masculine ones to the morning one. Some of the earlier civilisations of the Middle East regarded the planet as embodying both and portrayed it as a hermaphrodite. By the time astrology, as we know it, was being formulated by the Babylonians, though, the planet was firmly established as feminine and was associated with the goddess Ishtar. The Greeks called her Aphrodite and transferred her former masculine attributes to her son, Eros, while the Romans gave her the name by which we know her today.

By that name she is universally recognised as the Goddess of Love, representing the sexual attraction between male and female. Does this, I wonder, reflect her earlier incarnations as both male and female, their later separation and desire to be reunited? Whether that is so or not, without the sexual act there can be no fertility, and virtually every civilisation has a fertility goddess. Venus/Aphrodite assumed the mantle of these great mother figures wherever Greek or Roman influence reached.

The Graeco-Roman myths tell that Venus was born from the foam that arose when Cronos (Saturn) cut off the genitals of his father Ouranos (Uranus) and threw them into the sea, arising from the foam as an adult woman of great beauty. She was carried ashore on a giant seashell, landing at a place in present-day Cyprus where remains of a temple in her honour can still be seen. She was married to the smith-god, Hephaestos, but was serially unfaithful to him, most notably with Mars.

Being without mother or father, Venus epitomises the independent woman and independent women are often viewed with fear or at least suspicion, perhaps with some justification in the case of Venus; for she was capable of being a trouble-maker, not only in her love affairs with gods and mortals (her mortal lovers usually came to a bad end) but because she sometimes meddled in human matters with disastrous results. She was, for example, the original cause of the Trojan Wars.

Because of her great physical beauty, Venus has come to represent all that is beautiful and is seen as the patroness of the arts, as well as all things pleasing to the senses: food, wine, beautiful clothes, sumptuous surroundings, as well as with sexual love. And in astrology she symbolises all these things, as well as social enjoyment and the company of good friends.

The position of Venus in a birth chart tells us about the individual's response to sensuous pleasures, beauty and the arts as well as love and sex. The special affinities of Venus are with the signs of Taurus and Libra, and people born in these signs tend to appreciate all things Venusian, though the manner in which they do so is different. Taurus is an Earth sign, and Taureans often appreciate the good things in life very heartily; while Libra is an Air sign and Librans may express their Venusian nature more through a love of the arts. This distinction is by no means cut and dried, though Librans may show more fastidiousness and refinement of taste. Venus is strongly positioned in a chart when it is in either of these signs and in Pisces, but weak when in Aries, Scorpio or Virgo.

Venus is now the only planet considered to have this kind of affinity with more than one sign. Only those planets visible to the eye were known to the early astrologers and, of course, there were not enough of them to ascribe the 'rulership' of a single sign to each one, so the Sun and the Moon were given one sign each, and all the planets two. Since the end of the 18th century when Uranus was discovered, the outer planets and Chiron have come to be understood as having affinity with Virgo, Scorpio, Aquarius and Pisces. Possibly, as we learn more about the planet that has been identified beyond Pluto, Venus will relinquish one or other of her signs to the newcomer?

Plants associated with Venus are those the old herbalists described as cool and moist, the best-known being the Rose, which has been associated with her since earliest times. Others include Geranium, Palmarosa, Violet Leaf, Verbena, Yarrow and Ylang-Ylang.

Aromatherapy itself can be seen as connected with Venus, because of our use of beautiful-smelling oils, massage and the nurture of the body, as well as the use of oils in skincare; though there is, of course, a great deal more to aromatherapy than mere luxury and beauty therapy, and the healing facets of the art have links with both Mercury in his caduceus-carrying capacity, as we have already seen, and with Chiron, which we will look at a little further on.

★ Earth ⊕

The Earth is the next planet in order of distance from the Sun – the 'Third Rock from the Sun', but our home planet does not figure among the planets in astrology. This is because when we consider the other planets literally, observing them in the night sky, we do not see the Earth on which we are standing. When we consider the planets symbolically in a natal chart, we imagine ourselves to be standing on the Earth in the centre of the circle.

When we speak of 'Earth' in astrology we are not referring to the planet, but to the *element* Earth, in contrast to Air, Fire and Water.

Astrological Aromatherapy

Mars

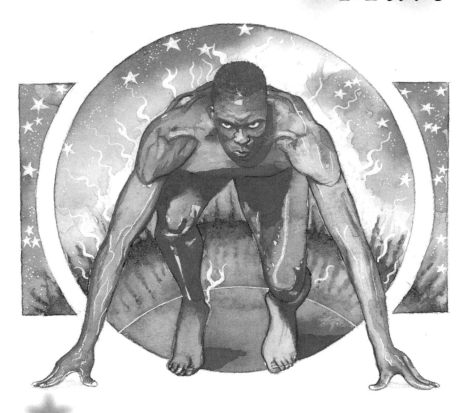

Fiery champion, warrior of spirit,

Giver of strength, source of our courage,

Teach us to use our passion wisely,

Lead us on in Life's adventure.

Mars ♂

Mars, the fourth planet from the Sun, is the first to lie *beyond* Earth in relation to the Sun. Perhaps it is because of this that Mars has always exerted a powerful fascination for humankind, as a stepping-stone to the stars, first in fiction and now in space exploration? The 'Red Planet' lies, on average, about 142 million miles from the Sun, though this varies because of its irregular orbit, which takes a little less than two years to complete. Viewed from Earth, Mars is a star with a reddish light – hence its name – which varies in brightness and size depending on whether it is on the same side of the Sun as we are, or on the opposite side.

In mythology, the planet has been considered masculine in all cultures, including those which had no contact with each other. Traditionally, the gods associated with this planet have been warlike – a fact that can be attributed to the red colour, thought to signify anger and heat.

The earliest myths associated with this planet can be traced back to Mesopotamia, some 4,000 years ago, when it was sacred to the god Nergal. The Egyptians identified it with Horus, calling it 'Horus the Red'. The Greeks named the planet Ares, after their god of war who was depicted as being clad in heavy armour and bringing death and destruction. His Roman manifestation, Mars, was a less belligerent figure and originated as a fertility god, associated with flocks and herds and male potency. In a predominantly agrarian society, he was a very important deity, for without a potent bull or ram the flocks would not flourish and the people would go hungry. Only later did he take on the warlike aspect of Ares, but even then retained his association with male sexuality as the lover of Venus, and the father of her son Eros (Cupid).

In modern astrology Mars represents the masculine principle in all of us, women as well as men, and the basic drive that enables us to respond to challenges of all kinds, whether they are physical, emotional or ethical. Mars is raw energy, the 'power pack' that keeps us going. Physically, Mars is linked to the adrenal glands, which give us the extra boost of energy that we need in demanding situations. Whether we choose to use that energy aggressively or put it to constructive use is our personal choice. The position of Mars in the natal chart gives us an idea of where and how the individual is likely to put that energy to work.

Something of the old 'warlike' associations still stick to Mars, but we can be spiritual warriors, we can 'fight' for causes we believe in whether they be our family, a political party or wider, maybe environmental, issues.

Mars has a special affinity with the sign of Aries, the Ram, doubtless originating from his early association with the fertility of flocks and herds, though of course the Ram with its head down and horns forward can be quite aggressive, too! Earlier astrologers also associated Mars with the sign of Scorpio, perhaps because the scorpion has a deadly sting and Mars was thought of as a death-dealing god. Although Pluto is now usually thought of as the 'Ruler' of Scorpio, the old connection still has validity, and Scorpio people do have tremendous reserves of raw energy, though they are often hidden, in contrast to the overt energy of the Arien. Mars is considered strong when in Aries and weak when in Libra. If you are ever in the National Gallery in London look at Botticelli's *Mars and Venus* which portrays this perfectly: Venus (Libra) sits still and alert while Mars (Aries) is totally vulnerable, naked, sunk in post-coital sleep while little fawns play with his armour, a perfect image of a planet in 'detriment' – to use the traditional terminology. Mars is also thought to be strong in Capricorn but weakest of all in Cancer. It is easy to understand the logic of this: Mars is essentially fiery and the profound wateriness of Cancer would extinguish its fire.

Plants associated with Mars are mainly those classified by the herbalists as 'hot and dry'. Many of them are tonic and/or stimulant, so valuable for people who need an energy boost, convalescents, perhaps for M.E. sufferers. They include Black Pepper, Clove, Coriander, Cumin, Ginger and Pine.

Jupiter

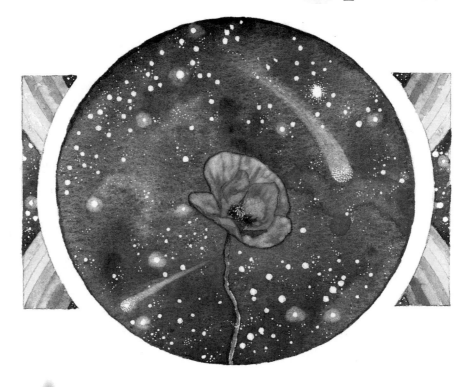

Bountiful lord and bringer of justice,
Sage leader of the ancient gods,
Teach us to give from our hearts' fullness,
Turn our minds towards the higher learning.

Jupiter ♃

Jupiter is the largest planet in the solar system, with a diameter 11 times greater than that of Earth. Its orbit lies some 484 million miles from the Sun and takes just under 12 years to complete.

Its size and brilliance led early civilisations to associate the planet with the most powerful of their gods: the Babylonians called the planet Niburu, and held it sacred to their chief god, Marduk, and believed that the appearance of his star brought good luck and prosperity. The Greeks, similarly, dedicated the planet to Zeus, the most powerful god in their pantheon. The Romans, inheriting the Greek tradition, called him Jove or Jupiter. He was the chief of a new generation of gods, having overthrown the powerful race of Titans who held sway before him. Himself the son of the Titans Cronos and Thea, he rescued his brothers and sisters, who had been swallowed by their father, and led them in a fight that resulted in the Titans being banished and Zeus/Jupiter and his brothers and sisters being established as the new gods of Olympus.

The name Jove has given us the word 'jovial' and that expresses one side of Jupiter's nature: he was expansive and bountiful, usually depicted as bearded and sometimes plump – almost a Father Christmas figure! His expansive nature also extended to his sexual appetites and, although officially married to Juno (Hera to the Greeks), he had at least three other wives before her and many amorous adventures with other goddesses and with mortal women, often changing his shape to gain access to them as, for example, a swan, a bull or a shower of golden rain.

He was also seen as the wise, all-seeing, just, law-giver. This did not necessarily involve clemency: he inflicted terrible punishments on those who transgressed the laws of Olympus and he sometimes let personal feelings supersede true justice, flinging his thunderbolts at those who had offended him. Thus he became, also, the storm-god, parallel to Thor in the Germanic tradition.

In present-day astrology Jupiter retains something of this dual character. It is the planet of good fortune and expansion, but also of philosophy and higher learning. In the natal chart, Jupiter indicates where we find our optimism and self-confidence, how we can expand our horizons and our religious or philosophical outlook. It may sometimes indicate the influence of a paternal, protective male, and also shows our own capacity for kindness and generosity to others. The negative side of Jupiter's influence can be a tendency to risky over-optimism, to exaggeration of all kinds and sometimes even to physical over-expansion, i.e. a tendency to put on excess weight.

Jupiter's special affinity is with the sign of Sagittarius and we find among Sagittarians many philosophers and teachers. It follows that Jupiter is considered strong in Sagittarius and weak in Gemini but also strong in Cancer and weak in Capricorn. In old, traditional astrology (formulated long before the discovery of the planet Neptune) he was also considered the 'Ruler' of Pisces, but modern astrologers, rather more logically, associate that sign with Neptune.

Essential oils associated with Jupiter are often warming and cheering, properties which share something of the expansive, benevolent nature of the planet including Hyssop, Marjoram and Nutmeg, but also some oils which have religious or spiritual associations such as Rosewood and Spikenard.

Astrological
Aromatherapy

Saturn

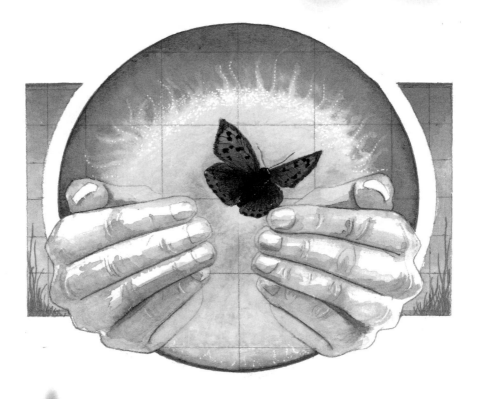

Old one, keeper of the boundaries,
Marking the cycles of our lives' unfolding,
Like a wise parent, like a stern teacher,
Help us to walk the path of wisdom.

Saturn ♄

Saturn lies 886 million miles from the Sun and has an orbital time of approximately 29.5 years. It is the second-largest planet, after Jupiter, and is the furthest that can be seen from Earth with the naked eye. Until the late 18th century it was considered the outer limit of our solar system.

The Egyptians identified the planet with Horus, the Babylonians held it sacred to the warrior-god Ninurta, and to the early Hebrews it was so important that they held their sabbath on the day sacred to it, a custom that persists to the present day with the sabbath being observed on Saturday (i.e. Saturn's day).

The position of Saturn as the furthest observable planet, led to it being identified as the maker or keeper of boundaries and structures, the one that held everything together. The Greeks named it Cronos and identified it with the chief of the Titans who was eventually overthrown by Zeus. They also credited him with regulating the measurement of time (giving us such words as *chronometer*, a clock). Even in Chinese astrology, which has a very different basis from Western astrology, the planet is called Chin, the 'Regulator'. Through regulating time, Cronos was also seen as regulating the span of human life and, as the keeper of boundaries, he was also seen as guardian of the gateway between Earth and the heavenly realms beyond. The apparently slow movement of the planet, taking more than twice as long as Jupiter to complete its journey through the Zodiac, suggested to the Greeks the slowness of old age, and Cronos was most often depicted as an old, white-bearded man carrying a scythe (with which he cut off life at the appointed time). By the Middle Ages he had become identified with both Old Father Time and the Grim Reaper.

As the Roman Empire succeeded the Greek, Cronos was assimilated into his Roman counterpart, Saturn. His feast, the Saturnalia, was celebrated in late December and was marked by a reversal of everything associated with the god: for one day all social boundaries were relaxed, servants became masters and vice versa; there was excessive eating, drinking, sexual licence and general mayhem presided over by a Lord of Misrule.

The idea of a Lord of Misrule persisted in England well into the 16th century – though with less licentiousness – when the social order was reversed for one day around Christmas time.

In modern astrology Saturn still represents structure and boundaries, but they are psychological rather than physical. Just as the ancients feared their universe might fall apart without Saturn's presence on its outer limit, so we can 'fall apart at the seams' without some structure in our lives. Saturn gives us staying power, self-discipline and the ability to take responsibility when that is needed. It also stands for old age, for the wisdom of the older person, and the position of Saturn in a chart may relate to an older person, an authority figure in our lives, particularly in our formative years – perhaps a parent or teacher. It may equally show where we are called upon to exercise authority ourselves.

Saturn is a necessary counterbalance to Jupiter, helping us to avoid excess, but if the Saturnian influence is allowed to predominate, we can become cold, hard, mean-minded and insensitive and, as a result, often very lonely.

Saturn's special affinity is with the sign of Capricorn and people born in that sign often show many of the characteristics of Saturn: tenacity but also sometimes a certain ruthlessness. Capricorn is where Saturn is powerful and Cancer where it is weak: just think of the Crab at home in the formless ocean and imagine what an uncomfortable environment this would be for a planet that represents structure. Saturn is also in a hostile environment in Aries – too much fire, too much change – but comfortable and strong in Libra.

The movement of Saturn in the sky brings it back to the position it was in at the time of our birth approximately every 29 years, a cycle known as the 'Saturn Return'. We can also observe times, roughly every seven years, when Saturn reaches points one-quarter, halfway and three-quarters of the way around its orbit, and these times frequently correspond with turning points in our lives. My personal theory (though I don't know anybody else who shares it) is that this clearly observable role of Saturn in the unfolding of human life could be what led earlier people to think of him as regulating time. Be this as it may, it can be very instructive to look at this cycle when planning aromatherapy treatments: is the person who needs your help approaching any of these Saturn 'markers' in their life? If so, what stresses might be manifesting themselves and how are they affecting that person's well-being, whether physical or emotional?

In relation to the physical body, Saturn's affinities are with the skeleton (structure) and the skin (our outer boundary) so it may be helpful to consider whether any Saturn issues are affecting people with skin or skeletal problems.

There are relatively few plants associated with Saturn. This may well be because early astrologers thought of it as an 'unfortunate' planet and associated it with death. The mediaeval astrologers called Saturn 'The Great Malefic'. Naturally, one would not want to link a medicinal herb with such an influence. Of the few that were associated with Saturn most were trees, often very long-lived ones such as Cedar. A more contemporary view of Saturn leads to the inclusion of Birch, Cajeput, Cedarwood, Eucalyptus, Juniper, Tea-Tree and Vetivert here. With the exception of Vetivert, which is extracted from a root, these are indeed all oils from trees. Another characteristic which most of them share is that they are all cleansing and antiseptic: Birch and Juniper are excellent detoxifiers and I identify these qualities with the disciplinarian side of Saturn.

Uranus

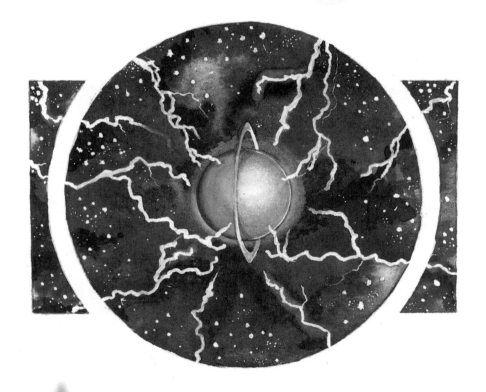

Wild one, bringer of the new, inspire us!

Herald of revolution, teach us

Not to fear change where change is needed

As we move into the golden dawn.

Uranus ♅

In March 1781 William Herschel, a German musician and amateur astronomer living in England, observed through his telescope an object which he initially thought was a comet but which was eventually recognised as a planet lying beyond Saturn, thus revolutionising our concept of the solar system. He named it the 'George Star' in honour of the king, George III, while the international community of astrologers preferred to call it after Herschel himself. But by the 1790s it had been generally agreed to call it Uranus, after a god of antiquity, in keeping with the other planets, though the symbol for Uranus still incorporates the letter H.

Uranus is about four times the size of the Earth, and lies in a highly eccentric orbit about 32,560 miles from the Sun. It takes 84 years to complete one orbit, and has an unusual feature in that its axis is tilted to such an extreme angle that, instead of spinning on its axis, it appears to roll through space on its side. This is probably the result of a massive collision with some other large body. Its colour is a clear greenish blue.

Ouranos (the Greek spelling of Uranus) was the god of the night sky, husband of the Earth-goddess, Gaia. They had a huge number of children, 12 Titans, three one-eyed Cyclopes, and several monsters. Ouranos hated them all – perhaps he had some premonition of his eventual fate at the hands of his son – and as soon as they were born he pushed them back into Gaia's womb. Gaia, wearying of this terrible burden, saved her youngest son, Cronos (Saturn), and gave him a sickle with which he castrated his father, throwing his genitals into the sea. (You will remember that Venus was born of the foam that resulted from this act.)

The significance of Uranus in modern astrology has less to do with the myth than with the observed eccentric nature of the planet itself, and the time of its discovery. I have used the word 'revolutionising' to describe the impact of that discovery on astronomy at that time, and it is significant that Uranus was first identified at a time of upheaval in world history. The French Revolution was only eight years away and the American Declaration of Independence had been signed not long before.

The anti-slavery movement was just beginning, as was the struggle for workers' rights. The Industrial Revolution was in its infancy, and scientists were investigating many new fields, such as magnetism and electricity. So the new planet became linked in people's minds with new technology, revolution, radical change, political idealism, intellectual freedom and original thought. Its eccentric orbit and odd manner of rolling through the sky doubtless inspired comparisons with eccentric people – especially by those who did not like anybody who challenged the status quo!

Such a correlation may seem simplistic, but it is entirely in accordance with Jung's theory of synchronicity: that is, that there may be non-causal connection between events that happen at the same time, that they are not random but happen at the same time for a reason.

Little by little, astrologers identified this planet with the sign Aquarius, with which it seemed to have strong affinities, and it follows that it is strong in that sign but weak in Leo. It is also powerful in Scorpio but not in Taurus. People born in Aquarius, or with Uranus in some other prominent position in their natal chart do, in fact, tend to be radical, original, nonconformist, not caring about the opinion of others and consequently may be considered Bohemian or eccentric. But it is their original minds that often shift our perceptions – the Uranian mind may be unpredictable but it can also be the mind of the genius. Such people can be very excitable and may look to aromatherapy for calm and relaxation.

I do not know of any plants that have Uranian connections. This may be simply because the traditional attributions date from long before the discovery of this planet, though many modern herbalists and aromatherapists have made connections between various planets and plants that were not known to or not used by their predecessors. Perhaps Uranus and the other outer planets are too far from our Earth to influence them? Perhaps we will eventually find connections between them and new varieties of plants? Genetic engineering comes to mind: a new technology that has revolutionised the way plants are bred. Maybe its products will be seen in future as Uranian, but I would certainly never envisage using essential oils from plants produced in this way as the potential dangers to individuals and to the environment are too great and have not been fully explored.

There is, though, one absolute, Violet Leaf, that I feel is very Uranian, although the Violet plant is associated with Venus. Other than that, when choosing oils for anybody with a strong Uranus (and it is strong in Aquarius, weakest in Leo) you might look to the plants that have traditionally been found beneficial for Aquarians, for example, Lavender, Lemon Verbena, Neroli, Pine and Patchouli.

Neptune

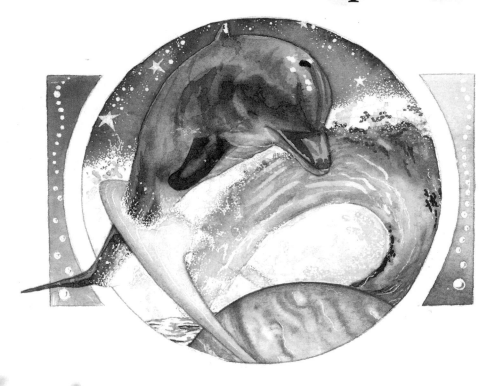

Dreamer of dreams and Heaven's mystic,

Shape-shifter, shaman, ruler of the oceans,

Teach us to know the substance from the shadow,

Lead us towards the realms of spirit.

Neptune ♆

The planet Neptune is about the same size as Uranus, and is about 2,793 million miles from the Sun. Perhaps we can better grasp the vastness of this distance when we consider that it took 12 years from its launch from Earth before the space probe Voyager 2 flew past Neptune and on into space. The great distance from the Sun means that it takes Neptune 165 years to complete one orbit.

The story of Neptune's discovery is a fascinating one: in 1845 a young Cambridge graduate, John Couch Adams, studying the deviations in Uranus' orbit, came to the conclusion that they were caused by the pull of another planet and, from this, predicted the position of this, as yet unknown, planet. The Professor of Astronomy at Cambridge did not consider it worthwhile to even check the young man's calculations. Adams went to London to see the Astronomer Royal, who was eating dinner and would not meet him! In the meantime, a Frenchman, Urbain Leverrier, had been making similar calculations, which he sent to a friend in Berlin, Johann Galle. The next night Galle and his colleague, Heinrich d'Arrest, found the planet where Leverrier had predicted. In fact, it had been sighted by none other than Galileo as long ago as 1612 but he had not recognised it as a planet and thought it was a Moon of Jupiter. So, who 'discovered' Neptune? I have related this at some length because, as you will see, elusiveness and uncertainty are typical of Neptune.

In mythology Neptune was, of course, the Sea god, or perhaps we should say the chief of the Sea gods, for there were others, including his son Triton. Sea gods are found in many creation myths, reflecting the primaeval origins of life in the ocean, but none of them can be seen as exact parallels of Neptune. Nothing about Neptune is ever exact. He may, for example, have originally been an Earth god, but by the time he appears as Poseidon in the Greek myths he ruled both salt water and fresh, the seas and the rivers. This made him a very powerful deity, for the rivers were a vital resource needed for irrigating the Earth, but if they flooded they could cause devastation, and the sea was a dangerous and often uncharted place. So, Poseidon was seen as an unpredictable god, one to be feared and appeased in case he caused great storms and floods or, conversely, droughts.

He was a brother of Zeus (Jupiter) and Hades (Pluto) and between them they ruled the Earth, Sea and Underworld...not at all harmoniously. Neptune quarrelled not only with his brothers but with Hera, Helios, Dionysus, Athene and others, usually over territory, which may reflect the fact that he had once been an Earth god and resented being confined to the sea.

Like his brother Jupiter he was a shape-shifter, and – also like Jupiter – he often used this ability to seduce goddesses, nymphs and mortal women.

When we look at Neptune in astrology, its symbolism is connected both with the ancient myths, as were all the planets that were known before the discovery of Uranus, and with the historical period in which Neptune was recognised as a planet. In the mid-19th century photography was in its infancy, with moving photographs, leading eventually to cinema, following a bit later. Many people at this time were fascinated by the occult and the afterlife. Sometimes this took the form of genuine spiritual searching but, equally, fashionable ladies attended seances or gathered in private round a ouija board. It was also a time when addictions of various kinds were rife, from the poorest of the poor trying to blot out their misery with gin, to poets and painters, such as Thomas de Quincey and Dante Gabriel Rosetti, hooked on laudanum or opium.

In this way, Neptune became associated with all that was elusive, illusory, not quite what it seemed, just out of reach. The shape-shifting god could be equated with cinema, for example. Addiction led to hallucination, spiritual searching might lead to great truths, but equally it might take us to the parlour of a fake medium with her butter-muslin 'ectoplasm'. So there are two sides to Neptune, the positive and the negative. This is true, of course, of every planet and every sign, but nowhere is it more true than in connection with Neptune. On the one hand we have the mystical, inspirational, spiritual facet which Gustav Holst expressed so beautifully in his music for Neptune at the end of the Planets. (The end, because Pluto had not been discovered when he composed it.) On the other, we have the planet of illusion, delusion and addiction. Neptune is present in all of our charts: how we make use of that influence is up to us.

The Roman poet, Manilius, associated each of the 12 Olympian deities to a particular sign of the Zodiac and made the obvious and logical link between Neptune and Pisces, the Fishes. Thousands of years later, following the discovery of the planet named after the Sea god, modern astrologers follow his example. Therefore we consider Neptune strong in that sign, as well as in watery Cancer, and weak in Virgo and Capricorn.

Neptune is traditionally associated with seaweeds and mosses and it is possible to get a Seaweed absolute, though this does not have any role that I know of in aromatherapy. It is used as a perfume ingredient, as are some mosses, so if you enjoy blending from a perfumery point of view, you might like to experiment with them.

Neptune is also associated with hallucinogenic plants but of course they do not form part of aromatherapy. We might look to Neptune in a chart for warnings of a possibly addictive personality, particularly if it is on the Ascendant, is weakly placed or has 'hard' aspects to it. Very, very few essential oils are physically addictive (and those that are, are among those that should not be used at all) but it is possible for people to become psychologically 'hooked' on a particular oil. To avoid this, be careful not to use the same oil too often for the same person.

Pluto

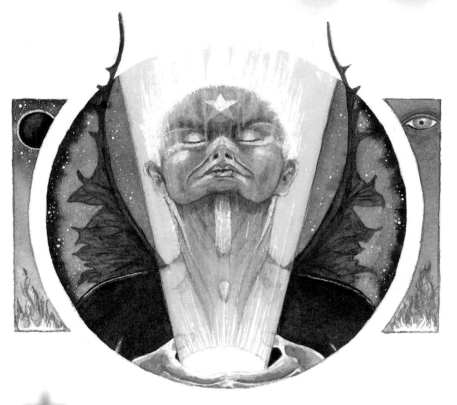

Dark one, ruler of the lower world,

Help us to overcome our fears,

Teach us that dying to the lesser

Leads us to rebirth on the higher plane.

Pluto ♇

The discovery of Pluto was, in some respects, comparable to that of Neptune, in that it stemmed from calculations based on the irregularity of the orbits of both Uranus and Neptune. Percy Lowell, a highly respected American astronomer, worked out the probable position of a still more distant planet, but died before it had been located visually. Another astronomer, Clyde Tombaugh, eventually pinpointed the planet in 1930, basing his research on Lowell's calculations. The symbol originally used to designate the new discovery was P, which could be read as either the first two letters of the planet's name, or as Percy Lowell's initials. Some astrologers still use this symbol (or 'glyph') while others prefer ♇.

The huge distances involved (Pluto is some 3,625 million miles from the Sun) made it difficult to estimate the new planet's size, though it was clear that it was smaller than Lowell had predicted. The ever-increasing power and sophistication of telescopes and space research has now shown Pluto to be even smaller than originally thought with a diameter of some 1,500 miles, only half that of Mercury, previously believed to be the smallest planet in our system. Some astronomers now query whether it is, in fact, a planet at all and prefer to call it a planetoid. Its very small size suggests that it is unlikely to be the cause of Uranus and Neptune's irregular orbits, and astronomers have considered for several decades that there is yet another planet waiting to be found beyond Pluto, and, in fact, in the autumn of 2001 such a planet has been identified.

Pluto's own orbit is irregular in the extreme, being more sausage-shaped than circular, and it takes the planet 247 years to travel round the Sun. In 1978 it was shown to have a very large moon, about half the size of the planet itself, which has now been called Charon, after the boatman who ferried souls across the Styx - the river between Earth and the Underworld. The idea that the departing soul had to cross a river was shared by many cultures, including the Aztecs and many of the Native American tribes.

The mythological Pluto was Lord of the Underworld: you will recall that he was one of the three brother-gods ruling the three realms of Earth, Sea and the Underworld. His entourage included the Gods of Sleep and of Death. His Greek name, Hades, meant 'invisible' and on the rare occasions that he ventured out of his own kingdom he made himself invisible by means of a magic helmet. The name Hades causes some confusion, as mediaeval and later writers adopted it to mean the underworld or hell, rather than its ruler.

One of the most important of the myths concerning Pluto is the story of Persephone, daughter of the corn goddess, Demeter. One day in spring Persephone was gathering flowers and picked a narcissus, a flower that was sacred to Pluto. The Earth opened and Pluto drew her down into his own kingdom to be his wife. When Demeter found out what had happened, she was so distraught that she failed to make the crops grow while she searched for her lost child. Eventually, Jupiter intervened and ordered his brother Pluto to release the girl so that his people would not starve. Pluto obeyed but, while she was in his kingdom, Persephone had eaten a pomegranate (some say that Pluto cunningly slipped a single seed of it into her mouth) and so she was obliged to return to the Underworld for part of each year, as anybody who had eaten the food of that world could never totally escape from it.

The idea that anybody who had eaten or drunk in the nether world was bound to it, is a widely held belief, and there are close parallels between the story of Persephone and the Sumerian epic of the descent of Innana. These myths are connected with the seasons, the apparent death of plants in the winter and their reappearance each spring.

As Lord of the Underworld, Pluto wielded tremendous power and commanded great riches, but it was power that was hidden, and in a natal chart Pluto is connected with our personal power, which may not always be apparent. Our greatest treasures may be hidden deep within us. Pluto relates especially to our ability to survive and recover from crises, growing and becoming stronger in the process. There are clear parallels here with the stories of Innana and Persephone.

The theme of hidden power is apparent also in the fact that the planet was first sighted around the same time that the atom was first split. Like nuclear power, Pluto holds the potential for good or evil. I'd also like to reflect at this point on the fact that each of the outer planets has been named by astronomers, not astrologers. Until not so very long ago, perhaps three or four hundred years at most, astronomers and astrologers were the same people but by the late-18th century, when Herschel sighted Uranus, the two disciplines had become separated and astronomers were very suspicious of astrologers. Even so, they have named each of the newly discovered planets in a way that has subsequently been shown to be totally appropriate to the astrological significance of the planet. Perhaps we can see synchronicity at work here, too.

Most astrologers now agree that Pluto should be associated with Scorpio, which was previously considered to be 'ruled' by Mars, so it follows that Pluto is strong in a chart when it is found in Scorpio and weak in the opposite sign of Taurus. It is also considered strong in Pisces and Leo and weak in Aquarius and Virgo.

There are, of course, no references to plants associated with Pluto in the classical texts because the planet was then unknown. I am inclined to attribute Cypress to Pluto because of the tree's symbolic association with death and rebirth, or eternal life. It has been planted around cemeteries for thousands of years because of this symbolism. Patchouli can also be considered a Pluto oil because of its extremely 'deep' aroma and its association with Scorpio.

Chiron

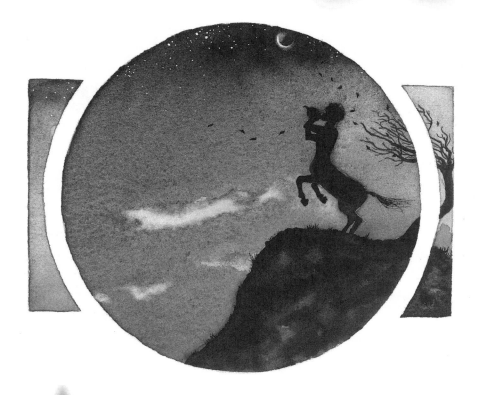

Healer, teacher we honour your great heart,
Wounded yourself, you salve our wounding.
Teach us, we pray, your timeless wisdom
That we, like you, can offer healing.

Chiron ⚷

Chiron was first officially identified in November 1977, although it was later realised that it was visible on plates taken as long ago as the 1890s and again in the 1940s. It is not a planet, but a large asteroid though, just as some astronomers believe Pluto is a planetoid because it is too small to be a planet, others consider Chiron to be a planetoid because it is considerably larger than most known asteroids and is possibly in the process of becoming a planet. Physically, Chiron is roughly a pear-shaped rock approximately the size of Wales. Its orbital time varies between approximately 49 and 51 years. The orbit is extremely elongated and swings at one extreme inside the orbit of Saturn and, at the other, that of Uranus. Barbara Hand Clow, author of the most authoritative text on Chiron, has called it "the bridge between the inner and outer planets".

Whether or not Chiron is a planet does not affect its significance in astrology, which is perhaps of greater importance to aromatherapists than many of the major planets, for its function is to do with healing and being healed.

Chiron is known as the Wounded Healer. In myth, he was a centaur renowned for his wisdom and was the teacher of other centaurs and of many young gods and heroes. He was also a great healer but he had a wound in his thigh which would never heal and, because he was one of the immortals, he was destined to suffer pain eternally. Jupiter eventually took pity on him and granted him mortality so that he could be freed from suffering.

Chiron is usually depicted as a man-horse, very similar to Sagittarius but without the bow. However, some Greek representations of Chiron show him with human front legs and horse's rear legs, emphasising the thinking, human, compassionate side of being over the physical as symbolised by the horse.

Although Chiron has only been known to us for a quarter of a century, its position in natal charts and its correlation with individual lives has been so widely studied that there can be little doubt about its significance. Chiron's position in the chart shows us where we have been wounded, and where the potential for healing may be found. We can see in its glyph a resemblance to a key and we may think of Chiron as the key to our healing.

For example, Chiron in the fourth house, which relates to the home and the experience of mothering, suggests that there may have been separation from one or both parents at a vulnerable age, or that the person may have been deeply affected by a change of home in childhood. Sometimes when we see a fourth house Chiron one of the individual's parents was a doctor or a healer. It could also relate to the experience of being a mother, perhaps to miscarriage or the death of a child. Equally, as Chiron shows us where the potential for healing lies, it may be that a nurturing home life will be the experience that brings healing to this person. Chiron in the seventh house of partnerships may indicate the origin of stress or even physical disease in a broken or traumatic relationship. If we have some guidance as to where a problem stems from, even though it may be a long way in a person's past, we are better equipped to find the best way of helping. You can follow this train of thought through the various Houses in the relevant section of this book.

In some people's charts, Chiron may point to that person's potential to be a healer or to work in a healing profession. Chiron in the sixth house, or in Virgo, both of which are associated with health and with service, figures in the charts of many therapists. Although there are some astrologers who do not include Chiron in charts, those who do are mainly agreed that its closest affinity is with Virgo. Therefore we consider Chiron to be strong in Virgo and weak in Pisces.

If Chiron is conjunct with a planet in the birth chart, think about what that planet symbolises: this can tell you much about the nature of the 'wound'. For example, Chiron conjunct the Moon can indicate issues around a lack of nurture: perhaps this person was separated from their mother at a vulnerable age, through death, illness, divorce or other trauma, or perhaps their mother was detached and seemed uncaring.

Chiron conjunct Moon often coincides with eating disorders in adolescence or adult life: anorexia is often seen as a desperate endeavour to gain attention from a parent, while overeating, especially when this is for comfort, may well be an unconscious attempt to get the nurture that was lacking in childhood.

It's also intriguing to note the timing of the discovery of Chiron: just as the significance of Uranus, Neptune and Pluto can be related to society and events around the time of their first sighting, Chiron was first identified at a time when interest in alternative therapies was becoming widespread, in particular, the holistic approach to health, which includes the whole human being (mind, body and spirit), when considering health and dis-ease. Chiron's orbit, bridging those of Saturn and Uranus, is significant here if we remember that Saturn represents structure, the physical body, and Uranus represents that which is beyond the physical.

Some astrologers have a theory that new planets are discovered at the time when humanity is ready for them. We can also look at Jung's theory of synchronicity: certain events happen at the same time because they are in keeping with the spirit of that time.

As far as plants and essential oils are concerned, I have not been able to identify any individual links with Chiron. I think it is more likely that the Wounded Healer is associated with all healing plants.

★ THE ASTEROID GODDESSES

As well as Chiron, a number of other named asteroids are now being incorporated into birth charts and used interpretively by astrologers. Of these, the four best-known symbolise four of the goddesses of antiquity: Pallas Athene (Minerva), Hera (Juno), Hestia (Vesta) and Ceres (Demeter). I don't propose to look at these in detail here because, unlike Chiron, there is not yet a sufficient body of evidence to show how they function in a natal chart. Suffice it to say that they symbolise, respectively, the virgin Goddess of Wisdom, the faithful wife or partner, the Goddess of the Hearth, and the nurturing Mother

Goddess, and you may find it interesting to look at those elements in individual charts.

★ LOOKING TO THE FUTURE

What of the future? As we have seen, astronomers have believed for some time that there is another planet beyond Pluto and, as I write in the autumn of the year 2001, news is arriving that a 'new' planet has, in fact, been identified by astronomers at the Lowell Observatory in Arizona. They do not yet have all the relevant data but we know already that it is large enough to be considered a true planet, not an asteroid, and that its orbit seems to follow that of Pluto, though it may take one and a half times as long as Pluto's to complete. At present the planet is known merely as KX76 but in due course the International Astronomical Union will meet to decide upon a name.

What its significance may be, how we may incorporate it into the existing body of astrology and what meaning it may have for aromatherapists and other healers, we cannot yet imagine. Neither can we know whether there are still more planets beyond that waiting for us to find them. But as space exploration and more and more sophisticated telescopes continue to evolve, it is possible that the boundaries of our solar system will be extended still further as other heavenly bodies are discovered. What we can be sure of is that if there are more planets than we now know, they will reveal themselves to us when we are ready to work with them.

A walk round the houses

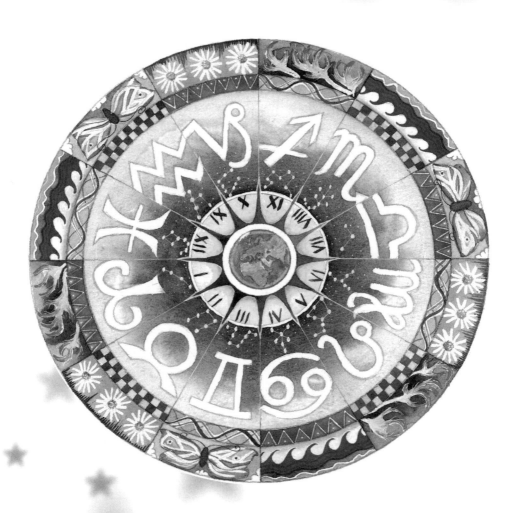

A walk round the houses

In the chapter examining the birth chart, I mentioned that a chart is divided into another set of 12 sections in addition to those that represent the signs. This second set of divisions is known as the Houses.

Houses in the chart represent different areas of life experience: work, play, home, relationships, education, career and so on. The sign in which a house falls will tell us something about the way an individual experiences that area of life. A house may have one or more planets in it, or none, and the position of a planet in a particular house can tell us how the individual is likely to behave in relation to that area of life.

For example, let's imagine that 'X' has Uranus in the house corresponding to career: Uranus symbolises everything that is new, revolutionary, unconventional, so we may expect this person to feel most at home working with new ideas or experimental technology, or approaching the whole question of career in an unconventional way, perhaps making abrupt changes of career when least expected. Such a person would be very unhappy in a highly structured, regimented setting such as the civil service or banking, whereas a person with Saturn in that house would feel quite at home in those circumstances.

Frustrations caused by being in the wrong job, being the square peg in a round hole, can be at the root of a great deal of stress and that in turn can be the cause of real, physical illness, so this is an area where an understanding of the birth chart may help you to formulate the most appropriate approach in aromatherapy – and this is an example applying to only one house, a single area of life experience. Stresses can, of course, stem from any or all of our areas of experience, so imagine this example multiplied by 12 and you can see yet another way in which the birth chart can be used as a guide to understanding stress, the causes of stress and possible ways to help.

Just as there are affinities between signs and planets, each house is also associated with both a sign and planet. In each case, the character, the 'flavour' if you like, of the sign has some connection with the area of life represented by the house. The planet, in each case, is that associated with the sign.

This is easy to understand if we consider something called the 'Natural Zodiac'. This is a schematic chart in which the Ascendant and first house begin at 0º Aries and the houses follow in numerical order, each occupying 30º, so that every one corresponds exactly to one sign of the Zodiac. Into this we can place the planets according to their affinity with the individual signs.

The Natural Zodiac is simply a way of showing these connections. It is NOT a 'real' birth chart: it would be impossible for any individual to have every house in its related sign and the associated planet in that sign, too. It *is* possible for a person with their Ascendant at 0º Aries to have each house corresponding to its related sign (if we calculate their chart according to the Equal House System, of which more in a moment), but this is uncommon.

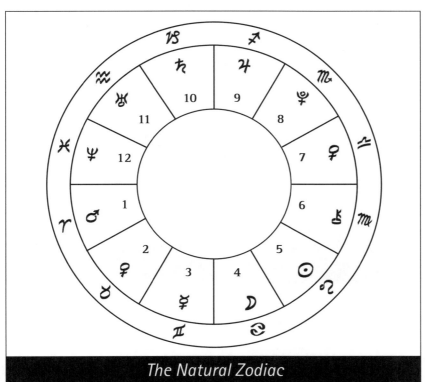

The Natural Zodiac

Whichever system of house division we use, the houses start at the Ascendant, which marks the beginning of the first house, and are read around the chart in an anticlockwise direction.

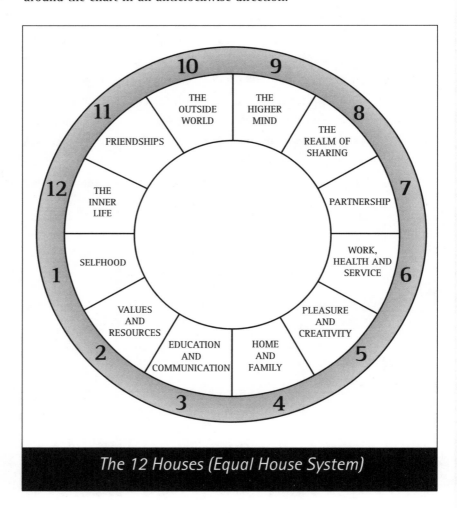

The 12 Houses (Equal House System)

★ THE FIRST HOUSE: SELFHOOD

Starting with the moment of birth, as marked on the chart by the Ascendant, we find the first house. This is concerned with ourselves, our primary experience of life, our self-image and how we learn to establish ourselves as people in our own right. It may also give an indication of our body-type, but this is not infallible. One way of understanding the first house is to think of a baby, the impression that the world makes on this new being, and that the new being makes on its immediate environment, then how the young child develops as an individual. This is a valid interpretation of this house, and we can follow through the other 11 in sequence looking at the chronological unfolding of a life from birth to death. That is only part of the story, though, because each house has some significance at every phase in our lives, and perhaps this is more true of the first house than any of the others, as it concerns our own Selfhood.

Looking at the affinities between houses, signs and planets, we can see that Mars gives us the energy to move forward through life, and Aries, with its emphasis on exploring new experiences, is very akin to the nature of early childhood.

★ THE SECOND HOUSE: VALUES AND RESOURCES

The second house represents the resources with which we are endowed and the value we attach to them, including our physical body which is our first and most important resource. Long ago, this house was associated with cattle, land, food – the resources that early people needed to survive – and represented security. Nowadays, we have a wider interpretation. For some people this house will represent property, money or other tangible, worldly goods, while for others it may be skills and talents. Anything which helps us to feel secure or to which we feel attached is a second house matter, whether it is an old toy we keep for sentimental reasons or the size of our bank balance. This extends to people, too, those to whom we become attached. Jealousy and possessiveness can be second house issues, if we try to cling to people as if we own them.

Earthy Taurus and its planet, Venus, have a natural connection with this house through their emphasis on assets and values.

★ THE THIRD HOUSE: EDUCATION AND COMMUNICATION

If we look at the houses in relation to the different phases of human life, the third house relates to our early years, to starting school and our early education. Even before we begin school, we learn to talk, in other words, to communicate, and this is also the house of communication. There is a connection between this house and the lungs, too – without breath we cannot speak. Saturn in the third house may indicate a tendency to asthma, so if you notice this in a chart you may want to ask about asthma or other respiratory problems. As well as the way we express ourselves, this house also relates to the way we take in information, communication being a two-way process. It is particularly relevant to the early stages of learning – higher education is something we will look at in connection with the ninth house. Remember, too, that we also use the word 'communications' to describe transport systems, and you will see how, by extension, this house also relates to short journeys.

The mentally orientated Gemini and its planet, Mercury, are both intrinsically bound up with communication and education in just the same way as this house.

★ THE FOURTH HOUSE: HOME AND FAMILY

The beginning (or cusp) of the fourth house coincides with the I.C., the lowest point of the chart, and it represents where we feel secure, the place where we 'belong', our home and the experience of family life and mothering. This relates both to our childhood when we receive nurture, and to adulthood when we may in turn become the nurturer. It is customary to use the term 'mothering' in relation to this house, and this may refer to our biological mother (or to ourselves if we bear children), but of course it may be either parent, a mother-substitute, or somebody else who creates the sense of security that a child needs to develop into a confident person. The way in which we experience the fourth house as a child colours the way we approach home and family issues as an adult.

The fourth house is concerned with our 'inner home' too, the source of our inner peace – or lack of it. For some people, this may be linked to their physical environment, while for others their surroundings will be irrelevant to finding that peace of spirit.

This house, emphasising home and family, is the natural place for Cancer, the 'mothering' sign, and the Moon which often symbolises our physical mother.

★ THE FIFTH HOUSE: PLEASURE AND CREATIVITY

The fifth house is not so easy to describe, for it bundles together a number of things that we might think of as disparate: love affairs, sport, children, creativity and entertainment. There is an underlying theme, though, and it is pleasure. This originated in the old view of this house as relating to whatever we enjoyed in our leisure time (as opposed to the next house which is concerned with work). Love affairs are fun – at least, we embark on them in the hope that they will bring us pleasure. Sport and entertainment are fun. This old way of seeing the fifth house also thought of the creative arts as fun, i.e. hobbies, leisure pursuits, though this might anger serious artists who know that a lot of hard work is involved. I prefer to focus more on the idea of creativity: we might not think our children are fun, especially when they are keeping us awake at night, but they are our creations, we make them out of our own bodies and they can bring us some of the greatest pleasure known to humankind. Conversely, musicians, painters and others often refer to their creations as their 'babies' (Degas, when a crusty old bachelor, always called his paintings *'mes enfants'*).

It's easy to link the outgoing Leo with pleasure and creativity (not to mention love affairs!) and the Sun, Leo's planet, with fun and leisure activities. Whereas the Moon-related fourth house connects with home and shelter, the Sun calls us outdoors to relax and unwind a little in summer; and even in winter a bright day lifts our spirits.

175

★ THE SIXTH HOUSE: WORK, HEALTH AND SERVICE

The linking of the themes of work and health also arises from an older view of the world: if you were well, you worked, and if you were sick, you didn't. Of course this is still true, but we also look at this house in terms of service. It is not the area of work in the sense of a career or vocation that is involved here (those are 10th house issues) but work as service. It may be paid work, voluntary work or the patient, day-to-day work involved in running a household, often repeating the same tasks time and time again. This house emphasises carefulness, attention to detail and usefulness.

Health regimes such as diet and exercise are also related to the sixth house, also the risks involved in overworking.

The sign on this house and any planets in it can sometimes give us an idea of what type of illness is likely, for example Saturn or Capricorn should alert us to the possibility of joint or skeletal problems, Pluto or Scorpio to urino-genital problems, etc.

It is easy to see how Virgo and the sixth house are linked by Virgo's patience and willingness to be of service: particularly in the caring professions, but not quite so easy to see how Virgo's planet comes into the picture, as astrologers are not all in agreement about which that is. Mercury is the traditional 'Ruler' of Virgo, along with Gemini, but many now feel that Chiron is more appropriate.

Certainly, when we consider the sixth house in relation to health issues, the Wounded Healer has very close affinities, and where you see Chiron in the sixth house of a chart there is a very good likelihood that the person concerned will be involved in one of the healing or caring professions. But the old 'Rulers' should not be discarded without a backwards glance – they can usually tell us something about a sign or house that supplements what we learn from a more recent attribution. In this case, Mercury tells us about intelligence and application to detail as it relates to our work.

★ THE SEVENTH HOUSE: PARTNERSHIP

The first six houses in a chart relate mainly to ourselves: how we experience our infancy, our education, our home, our work and our leisure. The seventh house is the first one which is seriously concerned with the way we interact with other people. The beginning of this house is always marked by the Descendant and, just as the Ascendant on the cusp of the first house relates to our first experience of the world, the Descendant directly opposite marks our first ventures into relating. This is the house of partnership. It relates to all forms of partnership: close friendships, business partnerships, marriage or long-term relationships, creative partnerships – wherever there is a one-to-one relationship seventh house issues are at work. In the seventh house we learn to co-operate, to give and take, it may not always be easy but we grow through the experience.

A person's best 'healer' or therapist can be indicated by the seventh house – this is another one-to-one partnership. What is it that makes us choose a particular therapist in preference to another, equally experienced, equally well-qualified? It is usually some aspect of personality that makes us feel more at ease with that person and, if we could steal a look at their natal chart, we might well find a harmonious relationship between their seventh house and our own.

Libra, with its insistence on fairness and balance, is associated with the seventh house, with partnerships of all kinds, and its planet, Venus, particularly with romantic partnerships.

★ THE EIGHTH HOUSE: THE REALM OF SHARING

Where the second house is concerned with our personal assets, whether tangible or otherwise, the eighth, lying directly opposite, is concerned with what we share. This may involve such literal sharing as a joint bank account or a house purchased together by a couple, legacies or trust funds and even such things as income tax. (We share our assets with the Inland Revenue whether we like it or not!)

But there is far more to this house than that: it is concerned with what we share at a very deep level, our sexuality and our emotions, both positive and negative ones. Pluto, Lord of the Underworld, is the planet associated with the eighth house, and much of what concerns this house is hidden, secret, taboo: we do not talk of our deepest emotions or our sexual desires, fears or experiences to any but those very close to us; sometimes we do not feel able to express them even to the people closest in our lives. Equally, we can see how the deep, passionate but secretive sign of Scorpio relates to the hidden depths of the eighth.

Pluto has only been associated with Scorpio and the eighth house in recent decades (the planet was only identified in 1930, you will remember), and before that Scorpio and the eighth were associated with Mars. The mediaeval astrologers referred to Aries as the 'Day House of Mars' and to Scorpio as the 'Night House of Mars', reflecting the secretive nature of Scorpio. Even though I believe the attribution to Pluto to be absolutely correct, we can see how the driving energy of Mars and its association with male sexuality can also be linked to some eighth house issues.

★ THE NINTH HOUSE: THE HIGHER MIND

This house is concerned with higher education, philosophy and religion or our choice of spiritual path. It also relates to long-distance travel, in contrast to the third which concerns early education and short journeys. We can read higher education in this context as referring, literally, to tertiary education: university or technical training, but also to the idea of philosophical, metaphysical or spiritual education. In the same way we can think of travel as physically journeying, but equally as mental exploration, the journeying of the mind, especially if this is of a philosophical nature.

The ninth house is a very natural habitat for Sagittarius, the sign of the traveller, while the planet associated with Sagittarius, Jupiter, embodies something of the philosopher or High Priest.

★ THE 10TH HOUSE: THE OUTSIDE WORLD

The beginning of the 10th house is marked by the Midheaven, the highest point in the chart. At the highest point, we are most visible to others (in contrast to the I.C., where we are private in our home), and this house is concerned with how we appear to people outside our immediate circle, our career, our status or role in the world.

In earlier times, this house was also seen as symbolising marriage, or the marriage partner, particularly in a woman's chart. This was because few women then led independent lives in the 'outside world' and their role was very much defined by marriage: 'the Doctor's wife' or 'the Parson's wife' for example. Now that women have careers in their own right, that connotation of the 10th house has all but disappeared. There are a few exceptions, though, where somebody (usually a woman) *is* identified in the public eye through association with a high-profile partner. Princess Diana of Wales is a perfect example, and her birth chart indicates this very clearly.

Capricorn, down-to-earth but capable of being quite ruthlessly ambitious, sums up a great deal of what the 10th represents in relation to career and status, and Capricorn's associated planet, Saturn, imposes the discipline and structure necessary to forge a successful career.

★ THE 11TH HOUSE: FRIENDSHIPS

This house concerns our relationship with the people we choose to associate with as friends, also organisations such as clubs, societies, political parties and charities – groupings of people who share some common interest. Often, this interest will be the achievement of some as-yet-unattainable goal, perhaps an altruistic one, for the 11th house is also the realm of our hopes and wishes.

The links between Aquarius and the house of friendships can be seen in the idealism of Aquarius, and the 11th house focuses on those with whom we share our ideals. Uranus, too, inspires idealism – you will remember that it was first sighted at a time of emerging democracy.

★ THE 12TH HOUSE: THE INNER LIFE

The 12th house is the most secret, the place of retreat, of contemplation, our dreams and the unconscious mind.

Where the ninth house is concerned, to some extent, with the outer rituals of spiritual practice, the 12th is to do with our inner life, which may or may not be connected with any organised religion. An old name for this house was the house of seclusion and it was associated with places where people were literally, physically shut away, including hospitals, prisons, monasteries and convents. For some people, a convent, monastery or retreat centre might be a physical embodiment of the 12th house, but for most of us it is more appropriate to think of this as the house of our most profound thoughts and aspirations.

In the cycle of life, this house can also be seen as symbolising retirement and old age, a quieter, more contemplative time after we have weathered the storms of life's ocean. We can see that Pisces and the 12th house share an affinity with the mysterious, elusive Neptune and the metaphorical ocean, the great unconscious in which we surrender our little egos at life's end.

★ THE HOUSES IN INDIVIDUAL CHARTS

However, as I explained above, the houses in a real person's chart do not usually fall in the sign that is associated with them in this schematic approach. More often, they will be in some other sign, and the sign in which a house *does* fall will suggest how this person will experience that area of life: for example, a person with Aries in the seventh house might be impetuous in forming partnerships, eager to explore new experiences through relationship. Somebody with a Capricorn fourth house is likely to value structure and stability in their family life, but might be a very authoritarian parent.

As an exercise, try to imagine each sign in turn in the first house: what would a Taurus first house be like, an Aquarius one, and so forth? Then repeat the exercise with each sign in the second house, third house, and so on right the way through to the 12th. Yes, that is an awful lot of 'homework!' but you need not do it all at once. In fact, it would probably be better to do this a little at a time, so that you really integrate what you discover.

Next, look at some real people's charts, observe which houses are in which signs and see how you can relate that to what you know about this person.

Finally, look at the planets and where they are in relation to the houses. For example, energetic Mars in the fifth house might indicate a person who throws a huge amount of energy into creative activities; but given that Mars also symbolises male sexuality, they might be putting all that energy into affairs! A 10th house Venus might indicate a career that is in some way connected with beauty: as an interior designer, a beautician or possibly even a catwalk model. I'm sure that by now to a large extent you will be able to work out the possible significance of other placings.

Now, what did I mean earlier by the 'Equal House System'? At various times in the history of astrology, people have devised different methods for calculating the position of the houses. The simplest and oldest of these, known as Equal House, allocates 30° of the circle to each house in the same manner as each sign. Later astrologers felt that this was *too* simple, that it did not reflect the fact that few of us attach equal importance to, say, our career and our leisure, nor do our experiences in the many different facts of life affect us equally. So they devised more sophisticated systems that allocated a different amount of space to different houses. The best-known of these is the Placidus system, although it has a drawback in that it does not work well for people born at extreme latitudes. The more recent Koch system, which also creates houses of differing sizes, attempts to correct this but still does not give completely satisfactory results at extreme latitudes. However, unless you are likely to make charts for people living in far northerly or southerly regions, Placidus works very well. If you are going to use astrological software, you will find that most programs give you a choice of house systems (mine gives 10, including some very obscure ones, and even that does not exhaust the possibilities!).

The houses do not, perhaps, have such a direct and clear connection with essential oils, physical ailments, choice of treatments and so forth as we can find in the signs and the planets, but they are still worthy of our attention, if only as an indicator of possible causes of stress. Mary, with a strong emphasis on the 10th house of career, may be miserable staying at home with her children, while her friend Jenny who has major planets in her fourth house, works in a high-powered job and worries all the time about her little ones being with a nanny! Both these women are likely to develop physical signs of stress (headaches, insomnia, allergies or digestive upsets, to name just some obvious ones) that could be helped through aromatherapy. If you have some inkling of what their charts say about these areas of their lives, you will be better equipped to help them.

The same holds true of every house, so do think of looking at these factors whenever possible.

Life cycles

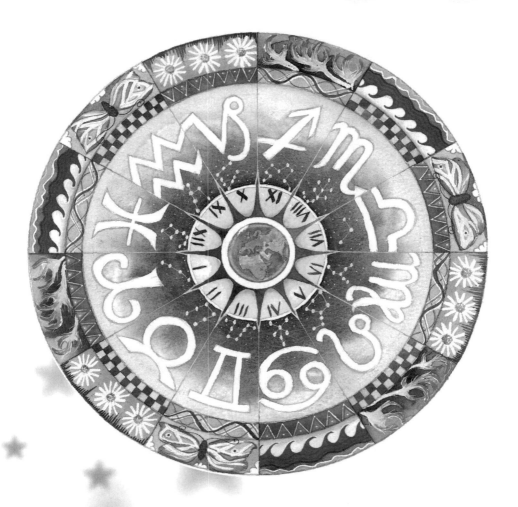

Life cycles

All the elements of astrology that we have examined so far have concerned the natal chart and what this can tell us about an individual and their potential strengths and weaknesses, both physical and otherwise.

There is far more to astrology than the birth chart, much of which is beyond the scope of this book, but there is one other area that is particularly relevant to the issues of health and healing, and this concerns the actual movement of planets in the sky in relation to their original position in a birth chart. These movements are known as Transits, and to understand their effect we look at where each planet is at the present moment (or at a specific time in a person's life) and the aspects that are seen between the planets in their present position and the planets in their original positions in the birth chart. The aspects, trine, sextile, square, opposition, etc., have the same significance as aspects in a natal chart. The possible permutations of such aspects from transiting planets to the planets in a natal chart are virtually infinite, given all the different natal charts in existence and the fact that we could look at the transits to any one of them at any moment of time within a span of several thousands of years (i.e. at any time for which an ephemeris exists).

The planets nearest to the Sun have swift orbits, so the aspects they make to the natal planets will be short-lived as they pass over any given point on the chart relatively quickly. As often as not they pass unnoticed and, at most, they may indicate a day or two when we feel less or more sociable than usual, a little brighter mentally or a bit slower, somewhat more inclined to lose our temper, and so forth. If you have access to an ephemeris or suitable software, it could be revealing to consider these transits when planning an aromatherapy treatment. For example, you might choose oils that are mental stimulants at times when a Mercury transit is likely to make somebody less alert than usual, or a calming, soothing oil if a transit from Mars suggests they could be a bit short-tempered.

The more significant transits are those of the planets from Jupiter outwards to Pluto. Because they have much longer orbits their transits last far longer, for several years in some cases and, because of the phenomenon of retrograde motion, will usually be experienced three times in succession as the planet passes forwards, backwards then forwards again over its natal position. The possible aspects that these slower-moving planets may make with other planets in an individual chart are too numerous to contemplate here, for the reasons explained above, though it could be very instructive to take note of them if you have access to the natal charts of people looking to you for help.

Even without access to the birth chart, though, we can predict the transits that the planets make to their own original position at the time of birth, and we can learn a great deal by studying these as these transits mark major times of transition in an individual's life. Such transitions may take place smoothly and, indeed, enjoyably but they may also be times of difficulty and tension and, as such, may underlie much stress. If we understand these cycles, we are better prepared to help people who look to us for help with stress and stress-related illness.

Taking the moment of birth as a starting point, each planet will return to approximately the same position it was at when it has completed one full orbit of the Sun (approximately, because the solar year is not exactly the same as our calendar year). These 'Returns' always mark some kind of new beginning in our life, the start of a new cycle. To understand this, think of your birthday: every year at our birthday the Sun is at roughly the same degree of the Zodiac as when we were born. This is our Solar Return, which marks the start of a new year in our life. That's what we are talking about when we say "Many Happy Returns".

Although the mechanism is slightly different, in that the Sun's apparent return to the same place is due to our Earth's annual orbit, the astrological significance is the same, and as each planet returns to its original degree we have a kind of 'birthday' marking the end of one phase of our life and the start of a new one.

★ JUPITER

Jupiter takes about 12 years to travel round the Sun, so every 12 years it heralds the start of a fresh cycle. At age 12, young people are on the verge of puberty, entering a major new phase of life as they move from childhood to adulthood. In earlier epochs, and still today in some societies, this transition would be celebrated with rites of passage. Nowadays, many 12-year-olds will be in their first year at a new school, which marks another kind of transition, but not so long ago in mediaeval and Renaissance Europe they would have been considered ready for marriage. For us today, the second Jupiter Return, at 24, often coincides with marriage or commitment to a serious adult relationship.

These first two Jupiter Returns may well be the most significant in many people's lives: the subsequent ones are seldom experienced as major upheavals. Jupiter brings expansion and opportunities and the Returns at 36 and 48 frequently correspond with increased income and status as people move up the career ladder. The next, at 60, will most often coincide with retirement, which brings the opportunity for a different kind of expansion: time to think, to read more, to explore new avenues and expand the mind. At these 'birthdays' Jupiter often gives us a boost of energy as a gift: a kick-start to get us going on whatever the next cycle may bring.

★ SATURN

The movement of Saturn in the sky brings it back to the position it was in at the time our birth approximately every 29.5 years. As this is a much longer cycle than Jupiter's, it is also significant to observe times, roughly every 7 years, when Saturn reaches points one-quarter, halfway and three-quarters of the way around its orbit. These times frequently correspond with turning points in our lives and, in fact, can be seen as corresponding to the 'Seven Ages of Man': infancy, childhood, youth, young adulthood, maturity, middle age and old age.

Somewhere around age seven Saturn forms a square aspect to its natal position, and at this time we are making the transition from infant to child. A square is a challenging aspect, and for many children this is a challenging time: they may be moving from infant to junior school, developing reading and writing skills and learning to socialise in a more adult way. At home, parents may expect them to behave more responsibly, help a little more in the home...and responsibility is a very Saturnian matter.

At 14, when transiting Saturn is in opposition to its original position, we are in the throes of puberty, facing all kinds of challenges relating to our growing awareness of the opposite sex, our education, our relationship with our parents and with society as a whole. This is often a time of rebellion, when young people kick against authority, perhaps as represented by their parents or teachers or the norms of behaviour that their immediate society expects.

At 21, when Saturn once again makes a square to its natal position, we are taking our first steps into the real adult world, perhaps leaving higher education or struggling with our first job. Saturnian issues around this time may concern taking responsibility for our own lives as we leave the parental home, or for the way we manage our study when we embark on higher education without the formal timetable of school life. They may centre on work and our relationship with our superiors there, while some people will already be taking on the role of responsible parent at this age.

The next crunch point in the Saturn cycle comes at approximately 28 to 29 when we experience the first Saturn Return. At this time we may be trying to establish ourselves solidly in the world, taking on responsibilities. It has been said that by the time of our first Saturn Return we will have experienced a 'taster' of everything that may come later in our lives, so this can be a good time to take stock and decide what we really want from our lives. We may look back at decisions we took in our teens or early 20s and conclude they were misguided and, around the first Saturn Return, some people make career changes or re-enter higher education. Parenthood becomes a major factor in many lives by the late 20s. Many people think of 30 – the Big Three-O! – as a major marker in their life, a time when they feel they have to 'settle down' and, if we look at this from an astrological viewpoint, 30 comes towards the *end* of the first Saturn Return, for the effects of a major transit like this from a slow moving planet, are felt over a long period.

A second opposition from Saturn happens when we are around 43, a year after the Uranus opposition when many people question the direction their life has taken so far and wish to make major changes. Saturn's influence at this time can help them to create a new structure for themself after the upheavals that are often involved in the Uranus transit.

The second Saturn Return, at around 58 to 59, often precedes retirement, and is involved with major changes in our lives. (Remember that, as with the first Saturn Return, around 29, the effects of the second will be felt over many months, culminating at around 60). For some people, the changes will be very welcome as they relinquish responsibilities and enjoy the freedom to study, travel, pursue creative activities or cultivate their garden. For people who have defined themself through their work, retirement can be extremely difficult. They feel diminished by losing their familiar role. Others may be restricted in their choices by a drop in income, perhaps needing to move to a smaller home or curtail activities they once enjoyed. Some will find themselves hampered by reduced mobility due to arthritis, osteoporosis or other ailments (remember, Saturn has an affinity with bones).

Occasionally we see people at their second Saturn Return making the kind of changes we associate with the first. This is more likely to happen if they failed to make changes they would have liked to make around 29 to 30, perhaps due to circumstances at that time. A surprising number of people resume their education as mature students around this time, often through distance learning, or turn an erstwhile hobby into a second career. I recall one woman saying she planned to use her retirement pension as a student grant to enable her to study music! Sometimes people who would dearly like to make changes in their life at this time but are unable to do so, for whatever reason, become seriously ill and a few may even die young.

Not all of us live to experience a third Saturn Return at around 88 but, for those that do, it marks true old age when we embody the Saturnian role of the wise elder.

★ URANUS

Once we move beyond Saturn, we are dealing with planets whose orbits may be longer than a human life span. Uranus takes 84 years to complete an orbit, so while those of us blessed with a long life will experience the return of this planet in our later years, others may not, and for the majority of people the most important transit of Uranus in relation to its natal position is the Opposition, which may be experienced as early as 39, though you will usually find 42 cited in books. Uranus's eccentric orbit means that different generations of people will experience this transit at slightly different times.

Uranus is the planet of sudden change, the revolutionary, the unexpected, and Oppositions, as you know, tend to be challenging times. It is no accident that this transit corresponds to the classic mid-life crisis. Perhaps we should remember here that the word crisis comes from a Greek root that means both crisis and opportunity. It is a time when many people make drastic changes in their lives: changes that may feel wonderfully liberating to the person involved and look like sheer lunacy to others. Have you always dreamed of selling up, quitting your job and sailing round the world? This is the time you are most likely to do it! It is the time when the high-powered career woman will ditch everything to have a late baby while she still has a chance, and the stay-at-home mother will go back to college or set up her own business. It is also, unfortunately, a time when relationships may fall apart, perhaps because one partner seeks change and the other doesn't, or because each wants changes of a different kind.

★ NEPTUNE

Neptune's orbit is even longer, taking 165 years to travel once around the Sun, so it will not return to its natal position in a human lifetime. Its transits are harder to define than those of Saturn or Uranus – which is totally in keeping with the nature of this most elusive planet. They often coincide with transits of the other outer planets in such a way that the impact of the Neptune transit may not be fully understood but will intensify the need for change at such a time.

For example, Neptune forms a sextile to its natal position at some point in our mid to late 20s, shortly before our first Saturn Return. Neptune dissolves and washes away. It breaks down boundaries, those very boundaries that Saturn has helped us to build, but in doing so it prepares the way for Saturn to create a new structure. A sextile often has some practical outcome. Neptune inspires our dreams and aspirations, and Saturn helps us to see how we can make them a practical reality.

Similarly, Neptune will be square to its original position in our early 40s, around the same time we experience Uranus opposing our natal Uranus and Saturn opposing its natal position. Small wonder that so many lives undergo tremendous upheaval at this time with three such influences at work within a short span.

★ PLUTO

Pluto takes 247 years to circle the Sun, so even half an orbit takes longer than the life of all but a few exceptionally long-lived individuals. We will experience a time when Pluto is square to its natal position but as the orbit is so elongated (more sausage-shaped than circular) transits from this planet do not happen in a regular pattern in the same way as that of a planet with a normal orbit, such as Saturn, for example. Was Pluto on a long arm of its orbit when you were born, or a short one? Depending on the answer, you may experience a square at very different stages in your life. Fortunately, it is possible to consult tables showing when this might be in relation to your year of birth.

Of all the major transits, a Pluto square is probably the most demanding. Huge upsets and transformations can occur at this time. Pluto asks that we look at our shadow side, experience our deepest emotions and learn from them. If we can do this, we will come through the experience stronger and wiser.

★ CHIRON

Bearing in mind that in this book we are considering astrology and aromatherapy hand in hand, perhaps the most significant of these major transits are those of Chiron, the Wounded Healer, for they highlight issues of health and healing.

Chiron has an orbital time varying between 49 and 51 years, and we all experience our Chiron Return around that age. For some women this will be associated with the menopause and for men and women alike it is often a time when we need to start taking more care of our bodies.

As Chiron is another body with a highly eccentric orbit, the squares and oppositions vary according to its position at the time of birth and can't be as easily predicted as those of Saturn or Jupiter, for example. As with Pluto, we need to consult a table that relates them to the year of birth.

As you may expect, the major points of the Chiron cycle frequently highlight issues relating to health and healing. (This does NOT mean that they are a portent of illness, although for some people illness may be the impetus for change.) If we take a holistic view of health, anything that affects us mentally, emotionally or spiritually as well as physically is a factor in our overall health. At times when Chiron is making a square or an opposition to its natal position we find that people often make changes such as entering or re-entering education, changing their job, or moving house. They may enter a different phase of family life, such as becoming a parent, or a grandparent, or seeing the last child leave home. Any one of these changes can entail a degree of stress, even if we have entered into them willingly and by choice. When we are pushed into changes that we have not chosen the level of stress involved is likely, of course, to be greater and our health may suffer as a result. Even small changes that affect our health, such as an alteration to our diet or beginning an exercise programme, are linked to Chiron and may well coincide with a Chiron transit, most typically Chiron moving into the sixth house or aspecting a planet in that house.

★ OTHER MAJOR TRANSITS

Other transits of the outer planets which may have a major impact on our lives are when they move from one sign to another, from one house to another or cross over one of the angles of the natal chart. The timing of these transits can't be predicted like the squares, oppositions and returns we have been looking at as they vary according to the individual chart.

When a transiting planet moves from one sign to another, its influence will be experienced in a new way, coloured by the nature of the new sign into which it has moved. For example, Saturn in Aquarius will feel subtly different from Saturn in Capricorn: in Capricorn, Saturn is in its 'own' sign, where its energy is at one with that of the sign, while in Aquarius it struggles to impose order on a more chaotic energy. We may experience this as an easing of restrictions (Saturn/Capricorn) or the ability to see a practical pattern or structure in areas of thought that were previously rather abstract (Saturn/Aquarius). These changes are usually felt most powerfully at the time when they are inaugurated, that is, when the planet involved is right at the beginning of the new sign.

Such changes are felt very strongly when they involve signs that have no planets in them in the natal chart, as the transiting planet activates some facet of our personality which may have been dormant until then. For example, a planet moving into Aries when there is no natal planet there may inspire us to be more adventurous, while one moving into an empty Libra could increase our involvement in partnerships.

Jupiter moves into a new sign roughly once a year, journeying through the whole Zodiac as it completes its 12-year orbit. Saturn spends about two and a half years in each sign, while Uranus will stay in the same sign for about seven years before moving into the next so that we will only experience its influence in all the signs if we live to 84 or beyond. Neptune spends about 13 years in each sign, so its influence will only be felt in half of the signs, or less depending on a person's life span. When we come to Pluto, the extreme irregularity of its orbit means that the time it stays in one sign varies from about 12 years to as much as 32 years.

Much of the same is true when planets move from one house to another, though here the change in significance will be in the various areas of life experience that are associated with the different houses. The movement of a planet over the beginning (cusp) of a house will shift the emphasis in our lives from play to work, for example, or from career to friendship. Where a house has no planets in the natal chart, it is rather like a stage with no actors on it: the arrival of a new planet on the stage can mark the beginning of a fresh phase in the unfolding drama of our life. The timing of such shifts and the length of time each planet stays in a particular house can't be predicted as simply as the movement between signs as each sign occupies the same amount of space, i.e. 30°, of the natal chart whereas the houses vary in size (unless we are working with the Equal House System, in which case the houses will also be a uniform 30°). So the time a planet spends in each house will vary with the size of the house as well as the planet's motion.

The movement of a planet over one of the angles of the chart is particularly significant, and never more so than when it transits the Ascendant. Transits to the Ascendant mark the start of a new cycle: Jupiter on the Ascendant may bring increased finances or more opportunities for mental expansion, particularly in the realms of philosophy or religion, and it is often accompanied by a feeling of increased confidence, a sense that anything is possible. When Saturn crosses the Ascendant we may have to take more responsibility for directing our lives, or it may shift our experience of authority and boundaries. Uranus and Neptune are both likely to inaugurate change, albeit in very different ways: Uranus on the Ascendant can feel very exciting. We may take up new challenges but there is also an increased risk of accidents such as falls and broken bones. Neptune transiting the Ascendant tends to be disorientating, but it is also a time when it will feel right to take up (or resume) the study of music, dance or meditation.

Pluto crossing the Ascendant is often very painful and challenging. It can bring up hidden memories, maybe of painful issues from our past which need to be forgiven and healed. At such a time we have to be prepared to let go of everything, and counselling or psychotherapy is often very valuable. There may be thoughts about death, or life-and-death issues which we need to face and resolve so that we can move on. If we have the courage to do this it will lead eventually to feeling as if we have been reborn.

★ SOME REAL-LIFE EXPERIENCES

In order to understand how these major transits operate in real people's lives, it may help to look at some examples of life crises that confronted various people at astrologically significant points in their lives.

SONIA AND PETE

Sonia was nearly 21 and her boyfriend Pete was a few months older when she became pregnant. Both were studying for degrees and Pete wanted her to terminate the pregnancy, mainly because he thought it would be tragic for Sonia to drop out of university at that point, but also because he could see no way in which they could find suitable accommodation or manage financially. He also had a desire to travel, which would be far more difficult with a baby. Sonia, though understanding Pete's reasoning, was deeply troubled by the idea of termination and became very stressed, unable to eat or sleep. Her older sister introduced her to an aromatherapist and gave her a voucher for a series of massages as an early birthday present. Now, one of the first questions that an aromatherapist will ask every woman of childbearing age at their first visit is, "Are you pregnant?" so that, if necessary, they can avoid the use of any oil that might harm the foetus. So Sonia's dilemma was brought into focus within minutes of her entering the consulting room.

Over the next three weeks her aromatherapist helped her with calming, antidepressant oils and also, with Sonia's permission, drew up a birth chart which revealed that Saturn in her natal chart was in the fourth house, the realm of home and family and was conjunct her Moon, the planet most closely connected with motherhood and, at age 21, transiting Saturn was, of course, making a square to both these planets. Later, a look at Pete's chart showed his natal Saturn to be in the ninth house, relating to higher learning, also that his ninth house was in Sagittarius, the sign that most closely corresponds to the ninth, so from the astrological point of view it was understandable that he would place great emphasis on both himself and Sonia completing their degree studies, equally that he would have a desire for travel.

Once the couple decided to confide in their parents, both sets were immensely supportive (it would have been interesting to see their charts, too) both with finance and offers of childcare if Sonia wanted to go back to studying later. Pete was happy, in a sober kind of way, and ready to support Sonia in her decision to continue the pregnancy. Sonia negotiated a year out of her course and went back on a part-time basis after she had her baby – a little boy who was wildly spoilt by a fond grandma on the days when Sonia had lectures.

Both Pete and Sonia were faced with tough decisions as Saturn formed this square in their charts, and both chose to take on the heavy responsibility of bringing up a child and completing their education at the same time.

CELIA

Celia was one of my own clients. She was 41 when she first came for a session explaining that she simply wanted some massages for pleasure and relaxation. She was married with two teenaged children, had no major health problems and did no work outside the home – she had no need to, she said, as Howard, her husband, made "pots of money". (Her clothes, hair, jewellery and general grooming had already suggested as much.) I noted from her date of birth that Celia was a Libran, and I made a blend of Ylang-Ylang and Geranium for her massage. Both these oils are associated with Venus and were entirely appropriate to Celia's request for relaxation and pleasure. However, over the course of several visits at weekly intervals, I sensed an undercurrent of discontent, even depression, beneath Celia's *soignée* exterior, and so I made various blends including Bergamot and Neroli, but nearly always including Geranium, Celia's Signature Oil.

One afternoon, Celia arrived red-eyed and haggard and said she'd had a major row with her husband the previous night. I sat her down with a cup of Camomile tea and let her talk as long as she wanted before starting her massage. It emerged that Celia wanted to take a course in floristry at the local technical college and Howard had made fun of her for wanting to go to college at her age and at the same time as their son was due to start a degree course. He'd called her immature, spoilt and unrealistic and could not understand that she was not fulfilled by spending all day every day at home, where she had not even much to do domestically as they had a housekeeper who came in daily. "What he really means is that he just wants me to be around looking decorative when he brings his business contacts home for a drink or dinner", she sniffed. "He doesn't understand that I am bored out of my skull, with Gemma at school all day and Danny on the point of going up to Oxford."

Over the next few months, the situation escalated. I helped Celia as much as I could through aromatherapy, giving her oils for the bath, suggestions for blends to vaporise in the house as well as her regular massages. She decided to enrol for the floristry course, despite Howard's opposition, and this eventually triggered a monumental row. Just short of her 42nd birthday she announced that she couldn't take any more and was moving out with Gemma – Danny was already established in his student lodgings at Oxford – and had found a flat to rent in the next town, from where she could easily drop Gemma off at her school and drive on to college.

By the time a rather acrimonious divorce had been finalised, Celia was a newly qualified florist. By good luck (or synchronicity?) she heard that the florist in a small market town nearby was about to retire, and she was able to buy the shop in the town centre with two floors of living accommodation above so that there was adequate room for herself and Gemma, and for Danny during vacations. Celia blossomed, like the flowers she handled, and rediscovered a confidence in herself and her abilities that had been submerged during her marriage.

During this time of transition, Celia had Neptune squaring Neptune, followed by the Uranus opposition and second Saturn opposition. Neptune dissolved much of what had gone before and highlighted her dissatisfaction with an empty lifestyle. Uranus, the planet of change and freedom, emphasised her need to change what was unsatisfactory and be her own person, while Saturn eventually brought a new structure into her life.

STEVEN

Steven was also in his early 40s when I first met him so he was experiencing very similar planetary transits. However, as you will see, Neptune square Neptune had more significance for him than for Celia, while the Uranus transit had less.

Steven was referred to me by an acupuncturist who hoped that massage would help him with muscular pain. He was on extended sick leave from the high street bank where he was an assistant manager, suffering from extreme weakness, frequent muscular pain and bouts of vertigo combined with lack of physical co-ordination. His GP had labelled his problem as post-viral fatigue syndrome after a barrage of tests had revealed no neurological or other disease, but had been unable to help him apart from prescribing a drug to alleviate the vertigo. Steven had tried acupuncture, with a considerable amount of success, especially in boosting his energy and reducing the giddiness, but was still in pain much of the time, far from well enough to go back to work and understandably depressed much of the time, despite loving support from his wife, Mary.

Post-viral fatigue syndrome is a very Neptunian illness: it is difficult to define (some doctors would query whether it exists at all); the symptoms vary from one person to another, and so does the length of time it persists. If it continues for more than a few months, it might be described as M.E. – an equally nebulous condition – though every bit as real and distressing for the sufferer, who may feel that his strength is ebbing away.

Having noted that Steven's Sun sign was Aries, I realised that the weakness and the enforced inaction would be even more distressing and frustrating for him than it might be for some others. Ariens love action and their planet, Mars, epitomises energy, but Steven's present situation deprived him of both. Though, ironically, M.E. and similar conditions often affect people who are strongly Arien, usually because they have been driving themselves too hard.

Fortunately Steven's signature oil, Rosemary, is one of the first that would suggest itself for extreme fatigue regardless of a person's Sun sign, so I used that for his first massage in combination with Tea-Tree to rebuild his immune system, and Bergamot to help with the depression. He found this helpful, and we stayed with variations on that theme for some time.

Because getting to me for treatment exhausted him, even with Mary driving him to and from consultations, I offered to make home visits, and Mary invariably offered me a cup of tea at the end of each session. As a result of the conversations that accompanied the tea I got to know perhaps more about Steven than most of my clients. He had joined the bank at 18, straight from school, as a very junior trainee and worked his way up through the system. The bank had sent him on various internal training courses; he had moved around between three or four local branches and he was generally expected to be offered a manager's post before long.

For some years before I met Steven and Mary they had been following a spiritual discipline which placed much emphasis on the ethics of daily life and what they termed 'right livelihood': in brief, making a living without exploiting or being exploited, trying not to harm the environment and respecting all living creatures. It also involved not dealing in alcohol, drugs or arms, and Steven had become increasingly concerned that the bank for which he worked held large investments in companies that were directly or indirectly involved with the arms trade. However, as he told me one winter afternoon after his massage, he had no experience of work other than banking, and was afraid to rock the boat when so many banks were merging, closing down branches and laying off staff, and he had to think of Mary, their children, the mortgage and all these practical considerations.

Because I knew about Steven's spiritual beliefs, I felt it was appropriate to ask how much he thought his illness was related to this dilemma, and he answered immediately that he reckoned the two were totally intertwined. We talked about the possibility of career counselling, and by the time I next saw him he had been given the phone number of somebody who offered such a service. It took very little time before the counsellor suggested taking Steven's considerable knowledge of the banking world to one of the various ethical investment groups. Steven said he could have kicked himself for not thinking of that by himself – but when you are as depleted and depressed as he had been, it is not easy to make positive decisions. He was still not well enough to approach any of the possible employers in that field, but from the time he was given that suggestion he began to get stronger. He continued with both acupuncture and aromatherapy until he felt well enough to go back to work and did, for a time, return to the bank until an opening came up with a company of ethical investment specialists.

The Neptune square transit often heralds spiritual crises, and in this case the dichotomy that existed between Steven's spiritual beliefs and his working life was making him ill. The change he made was ostensibly small (certainly not the Uranian kind of change that Celia made in leaving husband and home and learning a new profession in mid-life), but made a great difference to his life. We might see the influence of Saturn here, too, in Steven's desire to maintain the structure of his family life and the family's finances even when he was very unhappy about the work he was doing: when Saturn opposed his natal Saturn he was able to put a new structure in place.

JESSICA

Jessica was 51 when I met her and had just been diagnosed with breast cancer. As you might expect, she was terribly shocked but wanted to deal with her disease as positively as possible. We talked through all the available options: surgery, chemotherapy, radiation, and alternatives such as acupuncture, dietary therapy and spiritual healing. She was adamant that she did not want to undergo chemotherapy or radiation if at all possible but would consider surgery if necessary. She had already seriously considered going to a residential centre where she would follow a strict raw-food diet and receive a great deal of other help in the form of counselling, visualisation sessions and other complementary therapies, and in this she had the full support of David, her partner.

At her next hospital appointment she told the consultant of this decision and, although he was not keen on the idea, he agreed that a three-month delay would not be life-threatening as the lump was small and no lymphatic tissue was affected. So Jess spent several weeks at the centre, and continued to follow the recommended regime at home. It was tough, but David and all her friends gave her wonderful support. After three months, there was still a lump but it was less than half its original size, so she determined to continue with her special diet, visualisations and regular massage and also decided to see a healer who was highly respected locally. After a further three months, the lump had completely disappeared, though her consultant insisted on three-monthly check-ups for at least the next year. She continued with a slightly modified version of her healing regime and no recurrence of cancer was found at her check-ups during that year, after which she was asked to attend at six-monthly intervals.

Like many people who recover from a life-threatening illness, Jess began to look at life from a different perspective: she had a wonderful partner, good friends and a really good relationship with her adult children, but felt there was still something missing. Eventually, she identified the missing element as music. She had had a brief career as a singer before she married, but abandoned it when her two children were born in quick succession. Her marriage broke up when the children were still very little and she brought them up as a single parent, only meeting David after the children had left home. David had suggested several times that she join a choir but she had been too scared to sing in public, even as one of a large group. Now she decided it was time to take that plunge and joined a 'fun' singing group that met at the adult education institute, getting a great deal of pleasure from the rehearsals and informal concerts. It was at one of these that the conductor of a small, semi-professional choir noticed her beautiful contralto voice and asked if she would like to audition for his group. She did so, successfully, and now sings regularly with them, often taking solo parts. Jess's life is fuller and more satisfying than at any time she can remember, even though she still follows a very strict health-maintaining regime and has to visit hospital once a year.

Jess knew very little about astrology, and nothing about Chiron until I mentioned the asteroid in conversation one day. When I had explained that the Chiron Return often brings an opportunity for healing not only physical disease but our whole self, she agreed completely that this was how it had worked in her life.

DON

Don never tired of saying that he was a self-made man, proud of the fact that he had built up a thriving business despite leaving school at 16 with three not-very-impressive GCEs. He'd drifted around for a while, alternating dead-end jobs with periods on the dole, until his late teens when he'd gone to work in a boatyard. Here he discovered both a passion for boats and a talent for working with them, and spent much of his leisure, as well as his working hours, on the estuary. By the time he was in his mid 20s he had saved enough to buy an old boat and rebuild it in his spare time, eventually selling it at a good profit. With the money he bought a bigger boat, refurbished it for sale, bought two more small boats from the profit, and so on, until he had built not only a sizeable bank balance but a reputation as a fine boatbuilder and restorer.

Almost all his friends were part of the yachting fraternity, and in his 30s he married Cheryl, 10 years his junior, whose father had bought a boat from Don the previous year. They bought a house with river frontage and enjoyed an expensive lifestyle, which Don worked even harder to sustain.

Four years later a massive fire swept through Don's boatyard and two adjacent ones, destroying every boat and the greater part of his equipment.

Don was, naturally, devastated but swore he would start again from scratch. Very quickly, though, he realised that he was badly underinsured, and that his policies fell far short of the replacement value of clients' boats that had been lost in the fire and, as a result, he was declared bankrupt. The house and most of its contents were sold and Don and Cheryl moved into a furnished flat in the town. Don, who was used to drinking quite heavily with his sailing friends, began to drink on his own, beer, wine, vodka or whatever was to hand. His moods became very erratic and his temper would erupt with little or no provocation. On a very black day he lashed out at Cheryl, knocking her over so that she suffered really bad bruising. Not surprisingly, she packed her bags and left.

Don's depression grew worse, even large amounts of alcohol no longer seemed to dull the pain, and he began to experiment with cocaine, using progressively more as he became more dependent. By now, most of his friends were keeping well away from him but Cheryl, although she had left him – largely for her own safety – was still very concerned for his welfare, and went to see him, taking her father with her for support. Between them, they managed to persuade Don to go into a clinic, and his father-in-law generously offered to meet the cost.

It was in the clinic that Don first came into contact with essential oils, as several aromatherapists were involved in the physical side of the detoxification programme. Jean, his aromatherapist, began by using detoxifying oils including Fennel and Juniper to help his body in the self-healing process, but at the same time she was alert to whatever clues might present themselves about the origins of his addiction. Jean hoped to use astrology to help her with this and already knew Don's date and place of birth from his clinic records. With this information she could make what is known as a 'Noon Chart', which would give her a fair amount of information, but if she could ascertain the actual time Don was born she would make a more precise chart, giving his Ascendant. Luckily, Don knew this, as it was something his mother had often mentioned; in fact it was something of a family joke.

When Jean had drawn up the chart, she also looked at Don's current transits and realised that he was right in the middle of a Pluto square Pluto. Because Pluto moves so slowly, Pluto transits take a long time to complete and a square of Pluto to its natal position may take a year and a half to pass. Because of the phenomenon of retrograde motion, there will usually be three points during that time when the aspect is at its most precise, and at these times the effect of the transit is often felt most acutely. It is not surprising, then, that Don's progress towards recovery, both physical and emotional, was slow with occasional setbacks but, with help from Jean on the physical level and his psychotherapist on the emotional plane, he did eventually reach the point where he felt able to return to life outside the clinic, with continuing support in the form of weekly sessions of both therapies.

Life outside meant starting again from zero. As a bankrupt, he could not start a new business, even if he had the means to do so, and he had no other skills apart from those associated with boatbuilding, but he heard of a yacht owner looking for crew and took the risk of applying, even though he knew the man would be familiar with stories of his drinking and drug-taking – many of them exaggerated. Don was lucky in that the man remembered him as an excellent craftsman, knew about the disastrous fire and was prepared to give him a chance crewing for a few months.

Life at sea suited Don well: physical work in all weathers was hard to cope with initially, but by the end of the season he was probably fitter than he had ever been in his life. Working as one of a team gave him a sense of belonging that he had lost and helped to restore his self-esteem.

Don continued working as a crew member on yachts and began putting aside money to buy another boat of his own. He spent time with Cheryl when he was on land and, although they were not living together, both were making a real effort to rebuild their relationship. None of this was easy, but Don felt that he had been given the opportunity to rebuild his life from the beginning and, as he said, "I was a self-made man before the fire and now I'm making myself all over again!"

Pluto transits, especially the square, force us to look into the darkest parts of ourselves, but it is also the planet that signifies our ability to recover after a disaster, and Don's determination to do so suggests that he had learnt Pluto's lesson, however tough.

ANNIE

Annie was born in a small Suffolk market town, into a very close-knit family who all lived within about 15 miles. From an early age she loved drawing and as she got older showed real talent and was encouraged by her teachers to apply for a place at art college. Nobody in her family had any involvement in the arts and her parents were not at all sure that this was a wise course for their daughter. However, at parents' evenings the teachers assured them that Annie had genuine talent and it would be sad not to allow her to develop it, so she applied for and was accepted on a

foundation course at a nearby college. After a year, she moved to London
to take a degree course which she loved and found very exciting. At
college she was attracted to a fellow student, Jerry, two years older than
herself and they got married when she was in her final year, by which time
Jerry was working for a large advertising agency.

Annie got pregnant almost immediately, four months before her degree
show, finished her course with honours but did relatively little work after
the end of the course because of the expected baby. Two more children
followed in the next four years and Annie found such contentment in
motherhood that she hardly noticed that she was not painting at all. As
they grew older she tried getting her brushes out from time to time, but
was so often frustrated by having to put her work aside to cook a meal or
collect a child from school or nursery that she gave up trying. Jerry, who
had been so charming, such fun to be with when they were students
together, was less enamoured of domesticity and often came home late,
pleading deadlines at work. He was a very poor manager of the family
finances: though he was increasingly well-paid by his agency as he
moved up the career ladder, there never seemed to be enough money for
holidays or the children's clothes, and he would become either angry or
taciturn if Annie asked for more housekeeping money, which placed an
ever-increasing stress on the marriage.

By the time their eldest son was in his early teens, Annie had become
severely depressed and her GP suggested that it might help her if she tried
to paint, which she did with increasing success, exhibiting and
selling her work in local exhibitions. Conversely to what one might
expect, Jerry hated to see Annie painting. His lack of support and her
insistence on continuing for the sake of her sanity eventually led to them
divorcing when Annie was in her late forties.

Life as a single parent with three boys was tough: Annie got
a part-time job and, ironically, stopped painting again through sheer
pressure of time. She found London life with no partner, three kids and
little money more and more draining and often thought about going back

to Suffolk. At one point she was on the verge of doing so, but she had one boy preparing for A levels and another for his GCSEs and was reluctant to disrupt their schooling at that point. So she stayed in London until the youngest had completed his A levels, when she finally made the move back to a village very near to her birthplace. At the time of the move Annie was just 59.

Her children loved visiting at holiday times and weekends, and she gradually made new friends and re-established ties with people she had been to school with. She asked at the local adult education institute about the possibility of teaching, and was able to start teaching several art classes there when the new school year began, which brought her a modest income and left her enough time for her own painting as she tried to build up enough work for a small exhibition.

The second Saturn Return, at around 59, often presents us with choices or issues that we did not deal with at the time of the first Return. At her first Saturn Return, family life won the tug-of-war, undoubtedly because the needs of small children had to come first. But when Saturn once again swung over that point, she chose to put her personal needs foremost.

At that time, she had also had transits of Neptune and Uranus over the Midheaven of her natal chart (these were not squares or oppositions, but happened to precede Saturn's return to its natal position). Neptune dissolves, breaks down old patterns, Uranus urges us to make changes that are necessary, and Saturn puts a new structure in place.

★ CONCLUSION

These very personal stories are but examples of the many ways in which major planetary transits can manifest in people's lives. Your experience may be very different, and the experience of people who are seeking your help through aromatherapy will be different again, but I hope that this chapter will have alerted you to the significance of these key points in all our lives and how often they have implications for health and healing. Aromatherapy and astrology both have a great deal to offer in the way of support to anybody experiencing a stressful transit, whether through strengthening the physical body or helping the individual to understand what is happening. Sometimes just knowing what is going on astrologically and having the assurance that the transit will end in a predictable span of time is all that one needs to weather the storm.

With all major transits, the most valuable help we can give is to stimulate and encourage the energy of the Sun sign, using the oils appropriate to that sign and its planet. It is the Sun sign that nourishes and guides us at all times, as the Sun does for the solar system.

Approximate time of Pluto Squares to 2025

Year of Birth	Position of Pluto (Mid–Year)	Square	Year of Birth	Position of Pluto (Mid–Year)	Square
1920	7 ♋	1975	1953	21 ♌	1991/ 2
1921	8	1975/ 6	1954	23	1992/ 3
1922	9	1975/ 6	1955	25	1992/ 3
1923	10	1975/ 6	1956	26	1993/ 4
1924	11	1975/ 6	1957	28	1994/ 5
1925	12/ 13	1976/ 7	1958	0 ♍	1995/ 6
1926	14	1977/ 8	1959	2	1996
1927	15	1977/ 8	1960	4	1996/ 7
1928	16	1977/ 9	1961	6	1997/ 8
1929	17	1978/ 9	1962	7/ 8	1998/ 9
1930	18/ 19	1978/ 80	1963	9	1999
1931	20	1979/ 80	1964	11/ 12	1999/2000
1932	21	1980/ 1	1965	14	2001
1933	22	1980/ 1	1966	16	2001/ 2
1934	23/ 4	1980/ 2	1967	18	2002/ 3
1935	25	1981/ 2	1968	20	2003/ 4
1936	26	1982/ 3	1969	22	2004/ 5
1937	27/ 8	1982/ 3	1970	24/ 5	2005/ 6
1938	29	1983/ 4	1971	27	2007
1939	0 ♌	1983/ 4	1972	29	2007/ 8
1940	1/ 2	1983/ 5	1973	1 ♎	2008/ 9
1941	3	1984/ 5	1974	4	2010/ 11
1942	4	1984/ 6	1975	6	2011/ 12
1943	6	1985/ 6	1976	8	2012/ 13
1944	7	1986/ 7	1977	11	2013/ 14
1945	8/ 9	1986/ 7	1978	13	2014/ 15
1946	10	1987/ 8	1979	16	2016/ 17
1947	11/ 12	1987/ 8	1980	18/ 19	2017/ 18
1948	13	1988/ 9	1981	21	2018/ 19
1949	15	1989/ 90	1982	24	2020/ 1
1950	16	1989/ 90	1983	26	2021/ 2
1951	18	1990/ 1	1984	29	2023/ 4
1952	19/ 20	1990/ 1	1985	1/ 2 ♏	2025/ 6

This table is based on mid-year positions of Pluto. If your birthday is near the beginning or end of a year you may experience this transit earlier or later. Consult an ephemeris or astrologer for exact dates.

Table of major Chiron Transits to 2050

Year of Birth	Position of Chiron (Mid-Year)	Square	Opposition	Square	Chiron Return	Square	Opposition	Square
1920	10 ♈	1938/9	1945	1952	1970/1	1989	1995/6	2003
1921	13	1939	1945	1953	1971/2	1990	1996	2003
1922	17	1940	1945/6	1953/4	1972/3	1990	1996	2003
1923	21	1940	1946	1953/4	1974	1990/1	1996	2004
1924	24	1940	1946	1954	1974/5	1990/1	1996/7	2004
1925	28	1940/1	1946	1954	1976	1991	1996/7	2005
1926	1 ♉	1940/1	1946	1955	1976/7	1991	1997	2005/6
1927	5	1941	1947	1955/6	1977/8	1991/2	1997	2006
1928	9	1941	1947	1956	1978/9	1991/2	1997	2006/7
1929	13	1942	1947	1957	1979/80	1992	1998	2007/8
1930	17	1942	1947	1957/8	1980/1	1993	1998	2008
1931	22	1942	1948	1958/9	1981/2	1993	1998	2009
1932	27	1942/3	1948	1959/60	1982/3	1993	1998/9	2010
1933	2 ♊	1943	1949	1960/1	1983/4	1993/4	1999	2011
1934	7	1943	1949	1962	1984/5	1994	1999	2011/12

Table of major Chiron Transits to 2050

Year of Birth	Position of Chiron (Mid-Year)	Square	Opposition	Square	Chiron Return	Square	Opposition	Square
1935	13	1943/4	1949/50	1963/4	1985/6	1994	2000	2012/13
1936	19	1944	1950	1964/5	1986/7	1994	2000	2015/16
1937	26	1944	1951	1966/7	1987/8	1994/5	2001	2017/18
1938	3 ♋	1945	1951	1968/9	1988/9	1995	2002	2019/20
1939	12	1945	1952	1971	1989/90	1996	2003	2021/2
1940	22	1946	1954	1974/5	1990/1	1996	2004	2024/5
1941	3 ♌	1946/7	1955	1977	1991	1997	2005/6	2027/8
1942	14	1947	1957	1980/1	1992	1997/8	2007/8	2030
1943	27	1948	1959	1982/3	1993	1999	2010	2033
1944	12 ♍	1949	1963	1985/6	1994	2000	2013/14	2035
1945	28	1951	1967	1987/8	1995	2001	2017/18	2038
1946	15 ♎	1953	1972	1989/90	1996	2003	2022/3	2040
1947	2 ♏	1955	1976/8	1991	1997	2005/6	2027/8	2041/2
1948	18	1957	1980/2	1992/3	1998	2008	2031/2	2043
1949	3 ♐	1961	1984/5	1993/4	1999	2011/12	2034/5	2044
1950	17	1964	1986/7	1994	2000	2014/15	2036/7	2045

Table of major Chiron Transits to 2050

Year of Birth	Position of Chiron (Mid-Year)	Square	Opposition	Square	Chiron Return	Square	Opposition	Square
1951	29	1967	1987/ 8	1995	2001/ 2	2018/ 19	2038	2045
1952	9 ♉	1970	1989	1995/ 6	2002	2020/ 1	2039	2046
1953	18	1973	1990	1996	2003/ 4	2023/ 4	2040/ 1	2046
1954	26	1975	1990/ 1	1996	2004/ 5	2025/ 6	2041	2047
1955	4 ♒	1977	1991/ 2	1997	2006	2027/ 8	2042	2047
1956	9	1978/ 9	1992	1997	2006/ 7	2029/30	2042	2048
1957	16	1980	1992	1998	2008	2030	2042/ 3	2048
1958	22	1981/ 2	1992/ 3	1998	2009	2032	2043	2048/ 9
1959	27	1982/ 3	1993	1998/ 9	2010	2032	2043	2049
1960	1 ♓	1983/ 4	1993	1999	2011	2034	2044	2049
1961	6	1984/ 5	1993/ 4	1999	2012	2035	2044	2050
1962	11	1985/ 6	1994	1999	2013/ 14	2036	2044	2050
1963	15	1986	1994	2000	2014/ 15	2036	2044/ 5	2050
1964	19	1986/ 7	1994	2000	2015/ 16	2037	2044/ 5	X
1965	22	1987	1994/ 5	2001	2016/ 17	2037/ 8	2045	X
1966	26	1988	1995	2001	2017/ 18	2037/ 8	2045	X
1967	29	1988	1995	2001	2018/ 19	2038/ 9	2045	X
1968	3 ♈	1988/ 9	1995	2002	2019/ 20	2038/ 9	2045/ 6	X
1969	7	1989	1995/ 6	2002	2020/ 1	2039/ 40	2046	X

Table of major Chiron Transits to 2050

Year of Birth	Position of Chiron (Mid-Year)	Square	Opposition	Square	Chiron Return	Square	Opposition	Square
1970	10	1989	1995/ 6	2003	2021/ 2	2039/ 40	2046	X
1971	14	1990	1996	2003	2022/ 3	2040	2046	X
1972	17	1990	1996	2003/ 4	2023/ 4	2040	2046	X
1973	21	1990/ 1	1996/ 7	2004	2024/ 5	2040	2046/ 7	X
1974	24	1990/ 1	1996/ 7	2004	2025/ 6	2040/ 1	2047	X
1975	28	1991	1997	2005	2026/ 7	2041/ 2	2047	X
1976	1 ♉	1991	1997	2005	2027/ 8	2041/ 2	2047	X
1977	5	1991/ 2	1997/ 8	2006	2028/ 9	2042	2047/ 8	X
1978	8	1991/ 2	1997/ 8	2006	2029	2042	2047/ 8	X
1979	13	1992	1997/ 8	2007/ 8	2030	2042/ 3	2048	X
1980	17	1992/ 3	1998	2008	2031/ 2	2043	2048/ 9	X
1981	21	1993	1998/9	2009	2032/3	2043	2048/9	X
1982	27	1993	1999	2010	2033	2043	2049	X
1983	0 ♊	1993	1999	2011	2034	2043/ 4	2049	X
1984	6	1993/ 4	1999/ 2000	2012	2035	2044	2049/ 50	X

These tables are based on mid-year positions of Chiron. If your birthday is near the beginning or end of the year, the transits shown may be experienced earlier or later: check with an ephemeris or a professional astrologer.

Astrological Aromatherapy

Plants and planets

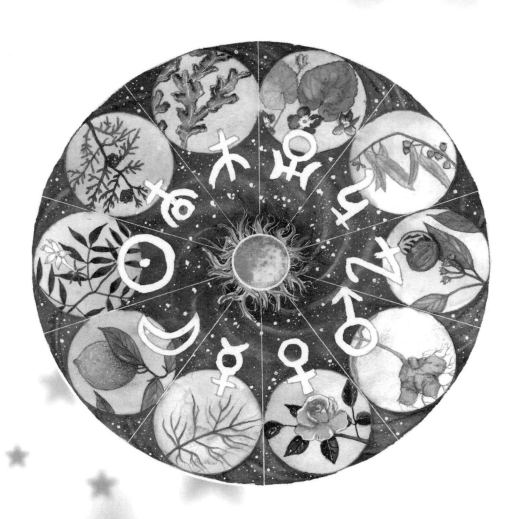

Plants and planets

When I embarked on writing this book, I envisaged that I would include a simple, at-a-glance table relating plants to the planets with which they were associated, but the topic has turned out to be so complex – and all the more fascinating for that - that it calls for far more exploration and explanation than a mere table could provide. I shall include some form of table because there are always times when a quick reference is needed, but the following chapter expands and examines the connection between plants and planets in more detail.

The most readily accessible source of information about plants and their affinities with the various planets is Nicholas Culpeper. He, in turn, drew on the classical authors, such as Hippocrates and Galen. But they all wrote about a great number of plants that we do not use in modern aromatherapy. Conversely, we do use essential oils from an ever-increasing number of plants that were either unknown to these writers, or which have not come down to us in the available texts. Another complication is that, in most instances, the classical authors were writing about the therapeutic action of the whole plant, whether fresh, dried or in water-based or alcohol-based extracts, but essential oils do not always have *exactly* the same action as the corresponding plant. There will, of course, always be very close parallels between the oil and the plant, but the latter may contain valuable healing compounds that are not oil-soluble, so the action of the essential oil will differ in some degree from that of its parent plant. In most cases, the difference is not enough to alter the relationship between the oil and the corresponding planet, but in one or two instances it is.

Further, we have astronomical knowledge that was not available to the old writers, not only about the existence of the outer planets, but about the physical nature of the other planets. We know that the Sun is not a planet, that it doesn't move round the Earth, for example.

So where classical examples are lacking, contemporary aromatherapists may need to make their own connections between plants and planets.

Some have made such connections and been brave enough to publish them. They don't always agree with each other, I don't always agree with them, and, invariably, none of us agrees with the earlier sources! I like what Scott Cunningham says about this in his book *Magical Aromatherapy*: "...the planetary attributions in this book are open to change if you feel the need. I've certainly changed them several times." So, if you disagree with my attributions, or anybody else's, do please feel that you can make your own.

So, how *do* we make the link between a plant and a planet? There are several ways of doing so, which would certainly account to a great extent for the areas of disagreement between authors.

One relates the growing cycle of the plant to the planet or other heavenly body involved: annuals were associated with the Sun because they grew from seed to maturity and then died in one year. As Mars has a two-year orbit round the Sun, biennials were thought of as Mars plants. Perennials were attributed to Jupiter, with a 12-year cycle, and trees to Saturn, which has the longest cycle (29 years approximately) of any planet known to the ancients. A variation on this system involves looking at the flowering or fruiting time of a plant, but this is less reliable as such times obviously differ from country to country and according to seasonal variations in the local climate.

Another system used by the classical authors involves comparing the known character of the plant with the real or supposed character of the planet: for example, plants that grow quickly and vigorously were often associated with the speedy planet, Mercury, hot spices with the 'fiery' Mars, more gently warming plants with the Sun, and plants with juicy leaves or watery fruits, which are often cooling in effect, were seen as belonging to the Moon, as were many white-flowered plants and night-flowering ones.

The appearance of plants would be taken into consideration, too: many plants with daisy-shaped flowers, particularly if they were yellow or orange, are considered as Sun plants because they are reminiscent of the Sun with its rays – Marigold is a good example – so were those with Sun-like fruit, such as Orange and most of the citrus family. Silver-leaved plants were attributed to the Moon or to Mercury by association with the silvery metal Mercury, and thorny ones to the 'warlike' Mars. The most beautiful flowers, especially pink or pinkish-white ones, were the domain of Venus. These included many fruiting species: almond, apple, cherry, pear, etc., reminding us that the planet was associated with nurturing mother-goddesses before the Goddess of Love. This system may not appear to the modern mind as particularly logical but it is no more illogical than the mediaeval 'doctrine of signatures' – and both 'work' in the sense that the plants involved do, in fact, have the therapeutic effect one would expect from their attribution.

Another approach was to look at the therapeutic action of the plant and link that with a planet. Just as each sign of the Zodiac is associated with a specific area of the body, each of the planets can be related to one or more body systems, so a plant that had a healing effect on a particular system would be associated with the corresponding planet.

Early writers understood the nature of the planets very much through the Graeco-Roman myths associated with them, and we should not turn up our 21st-century noses at this but be open to the insights the old stories can give us at the intuitive level.

I suspect that people who worked a great deal with plants and also had a profound understanding of astrology probably arrived at the right attributions as much through intuition as through the rigid application of any one system. My own approach has been to use a synthesis of the methods I have outlined above, giving precedence to similarities of character between a plant and a planet, and then examining whether the other systems support my conclusion. If in doubt, I have given my intuition the casting vote.

In the following examples you will see how various authors, both past and present, have applied these principles. Some of them will undoubtedly ring true for you, others may not, in which case, as I have already said, do not feel that you have to accept them blindly but try using both intellect and intuition to arrive at your own attributions.

★ THE SUN

Plants that are associated with the Sun include, not surprisingly, those which the old herbalists classified as 'warm and dry' such as Angelica, Benzoin, Cinnamon, Frankincense, Myrrh and Rosemary, and others which have something 'sunny' in their nature. Among the latter I would place Bergamot, Orange and in fact most of the citrus oils, which seem to embody the sunshine of the Mediterranean climates where they grow, Calendula and Helichrysum – indeed, Helichrysum takes its name from Helios, the Greek sun-god.

Culpeper classifies St John's Wort as a plant of the Sun and, although we don't obtain an essential oil from the plant, the infused oil is such a valuable healing aid I feel it should form part of every aromatherapist's repertoire. It is warming and analgesic and can give relief from muscular pain, fibrositis, rheumatism and arthritis – all 'cold and wet' conditions of the body – as well as minor burns, insect bites or stings and some skin problems.

It's worth considering here too that, in the form of a herbal tincture or tablets, St John's Wort is one of the best antidepressants available. It has been subjected to rigorous clinical trials and shown to be as effective as Prozac with no side effects and is particularly valuable for Seasonal Affective Disorder (SAD), which afflicts people in the dark days of winter when they don't get enough sunlight.

I have considered St John's Wort at some length here because depression is one of the areas that calls for Sun plants and, like the sunny oils, it is psychologically warming.

The Sun is particularly associated with the sign of Leo and you may well find some of the above oils appropriate in helping people born in that sign, though of course they will be valuable for natives of any of the signs, depending on their needs at any given moment. When Leo people feel that 'the Sun has gone out of my life' it can be very difficult for them to recover from the black mood that engulfs them. This brings me to Jasmine which I consider to be the signature oil for Leo. Various sources associate Jasmine with Jupiter, others with the Moon, but I have to disagree with them. Although the vigorous growth of the plant suggests Jupiter's expansiveness, and the fact that the aroma is more potent after dark could suggest the Moon, I feel that the character of the oil and its therapeutic uses align it firmly with the Sun. It is psychologically warming, one of the best-ever oils for helping with depression, especially with the feeling that this will never end, that there is no way out of it. It is also gently warming physically: Culpeper says it is "good for hard and contracted limbs" and in fact this use goes back as far as Avicenna.

★ THE MOON

Plants that are associated with the Moon are classified by herbalists as 'cold and moist', and are often night-flowering or night-scented. Many of them are not plants that we use in aromatherapy, but those that we do include Melissa and the various Camomiles. Culpeper says that the Egyptians dedicated Camomile to the Sun, but then calls them "the arrantest knaves" for doing so...without adding his own opinion! Camomile is cooling, soothing and anti-inflammatory, all properties that I associate with Moon energy. It is the supreme oil for babies and young children, invoking the role of the Moon as Mother. Melissa, another Moon plant, has very similar properties. Some people associate Jasmine with the Moon, presumably because the aroma is at its most intense after dark, but I would disagree, as I have explained elsewhere. Although the citrus oils, in general, are associated with the Sun, Lemon and Lime seem to have more in common with the Moon.

★ MERCURY

Mercury has an affinity with plants that are mentally stimulating, and those that have something mercurial about their habit of growth – either they grow very quickly, or have silvery leaves reminiscent of the metal, quicksilver (i.e. mercury). They include Basil, Caraway, Fennel, Lavender, Lemon Verbena, Myrtle, Parsley, Peppermint and Thyme. Several sources include Marjoram here – I'm tempted to disagree: it is a sedative oil but also very warming, and because of its wonderfully comforting quality I think it is an oil of Jupiter. All, however, are agreed on Lavender, the most versatile of all our oils.

★ VENUS

Many of the plants associated with Venus are those the old herbalists described as 'cool and moist'. They include most of the flower oils, and it is not insignificant that they are often flowers of great beauty, the best-known being the Rose which has been associated with Venus since earliest times. In Botticelli's masterpiece *The Birth of Venus* Zephyrs are seen scattering roses around her as she is carried ashore on a seashell. The Rose gives pleasure to the senses of both sight and smell, is traditionally associated with romance, and is given by lovers to their sweethearts. Rose petals were scattered at weddings from Roman times onwards, only being replaced by paper substitutes in relatively recent times. They were strewn on the newly-weds' couch, too, being regarded as an aphrodisiac. In aromatherapy Rose is still highly regarded as an aphrodisiac but also as a valuable treatment for menstrual problems and, as I mentioned in the introductory paragraphs, plants that are beneficial for the female reproductive system are usually thought of as Venusian. Culpeper includes Pennyroyal, Mugwort and Sage, presumably because of their action on the female reproductive system, but we must remember that he was dealing with the *herbs*, not the essential oils which are infinitely more powerful and all on the danger list. I mention them here only because it helps us understand one basis on which these attributions are made.

Other plants connected with Venus are Geranium, a balancer of female hormones, Cardamon, Clary Sage and Ylang-Ylang, all aphrodisiacs, and Palmarosa, much used in perfumery and skincare. Virtually all beautifully scented flowers can be associated with Venus, including those which do not produce essential oils: they delight the senses and this is another Venusian characteristic.

★ MARS

Plants associated with Mars are mainly fiery, those classified by the herbalists as 'hot and dry'. They differ from the 'warm and dry' plants associated with the Sun in that their action is often stronger and more immediate, something quite in keeping with the direct, even impetuous, nature of Mars. They are often hot to the taste or have a warming effect on the body, and include many of the rubefacient oils. Some of them are aphrodisiacs of the stimulant kind (rather than hormonal), and remind us that Mars symbolises male sexual energy. Many of them are tonic and/or stimulant, so valuable for people who need an energy boost such as convalescents, M.E. sufferers and anybody who is temporarily exhausted by work or other responsibilities. They include Black Pepper, Clove, Coriander, Cumin, Ginger and Pine. Culpeper includes Basil among the Mars herbs, probably because of its association with Scorpio, the sign that used to be known as the 'Night House of Mars': there may be an association with the word 'basilisk' here, as the herb was considered to cure the sting of poisonous insects as well as being used to discourage insects from entering a house. However, I think this is one of the instances where the quality of the oil differs somewhat from that of the plant and I have placed Basil under Mercury because it is a supreme *mental* stimulant and has somewhat less effect on the body.

★ JUPITER

Plants and essential oils associated with Jupiter are often warming and cheering, properties that share something of the expansive, benevolent nature of the planet, and also overlap to some extent with the properties of oils associated with the Sun. This has given rise to some divergence of opinion as to which planets should be associated with each of them: Culpeper, for example, includes Jasmine here.

I like to place Marjoram among the Jupiter oils, though nobody else that I know of does so. Culpeper, and most writers who draw on his texts, ascribe it to Mercury. One contemporary writer gives it to Venus, and I can understand that in terms of its warming qualities, but it is an anaphrodisiac, the very antithesis of what Venus symbolises. It is such a comforting oil, warming and reassuring that I cannot think of it as anything other than an oil of the 'jovial' planet Jupiter.

★ SATURN

There are relatively few plants associated with Saturn. This may well be because early astrologers thought of it as an 'unfortunate' planet and associated it with death. The mediaeval astrologers called Saturn 'The Great Malefic'. Naturally, one would not want to link a medicinal herb with such an influence. Of the few that were associated with Saturn most were trees, often very long-lived ones such as Cedar. Nowadays we have a less superstitious approach to Saturn and understand it as a valuable grounding influence. Consequently, we can associate with Saturn some of the grounding oils, especially those from roots which often have a dark, base-note aroma, particular those which are masculine in character, such as Cedar and Vetivert. I also associate certain detoxifying oils with Saturn, such as Birch and Juniper, and it is interesting that, although my reasons for doing so are different, this classification still accords with the old one of attributing trees to Saturn because they have a long life cycle.

★ URANUS

Very few plants/essential oils are associated with Uranus and even fewer, in my opinion, reliably. This may be simply because the traditional attributions date from long before the discovery of this planet, though many modern herbalists and aromatherapists – as we have seen – hold different views from the early masters, and have made connections between various planets and plants that were not known to or not used by their predecessors. I have seen Marjoram and Sandalwood attributed to this planet but cannot find the logic behind either. Perhaps Uranus and the other outer planets are too far from our Earth to influence them? Perhaps we will eventually find connections between them and new varieties of plants? Genetic engineering comes to mind: a new technology that has revolutionised the way plants are bred. Maybe its products will be seen in future as Uranian, but I would certainly never envisage using essential oils from plants produced in this way as the potential dangers to individuals and to the environment are too great and have not been fully explored.

One plant absolute that I would consider as Uranian is Violet Leaf, though I have to confess that the attribution is based mainly on the fact that Aquarians like it! It is, though, a rather 'offbeat' absolute and that fits with the Uranian picture. Violets, as flowers, are considered Venusian and Venus was born from the foam generated when Saturn castrated Uranus and threw his genitals into the sea. A rather far-fetched connection, I admit, but attributions have been based on less!

★ NEPTUNE

Neptune is associated with hallucinogenic plants, but of course they do not form part of aromatherapy. We might look to Neptune in a chart for warnings of a possibly addictive personality. Very, very few essential oils are physically addictive (and those that are, are among those that should not be used at all) but it is possible for people to become psychologically 'hooked' on a particular oil. To avoid this, be careful not to use the same oil too often for the same person, particularly if the position of Neptune in their chart hints at a possible problem in this area.

We can also make a natural connection between Neptune and seaweeds, and Jean Valnet found that seaweed and essential oil(s) together in a bath are more effective than either seaweed or oils alone, especially when there is a need to detoxify, such as in dealing with cellulitis. Various dried seaweeds can be found quite easily in health-food stores and through some herbal suppliers and I would certainly recommend using them in combination with essential oils where appropriate. It is also possible to buy a seaweed absolute which has some uses in perfumery, although I know of no use in aromatherapy proper.

We might also consider the subtle energy effects of essential oils as being linked to Neptune, for example when we use them as meditation aids or in off-body healing.

★ PLUTO

There are, of course, no references in the classical texts because the planet was then unknown. Pomegranate is mentioned in the legend of Persephone, but it is not a medicinal herb or essential oil. I think that Cypress, traditionally connected with Saturn, is more appropriately associated with Pluto: the tree is considered a symbol of eternal life, or death and resurrection, and has been planted around cemeteries for thousands of years for that reason. The Pluto myths are about regeneration so I feel this is a valid re-attribution.

It's possible that some of the very deep, base-note oils such as Patchouli could be associated with Pluto but with Pluto, more than with any other planet, any attribution is open to question and your opinion is every bit as valid as mine.

★ CHIRON

As far as I know, no individual plants are associated with Chiron: rather we think of Chiron as overlighting the whole of healing.

★ PLANETS AND PLANTS - A SUMMARY

SUN

Angelica, Bay Laurel, Benzoin, Bergamot, Calendula, Elemi, Frankincense, Grapefruit, Helichrysum, Jasmine, Mandarin, Mimosa, Myrrh, Orange, Rosemary.

MOON
Camomiles, Citronella, Lemon, Lime, Melissa, Petitgrain.

MERCURY
Basil, Caraway, Carrot, Fennel, Lavender, Myrtle, Parsley, Peppermint, Thyme.

VENUS
Cardamon, Clary Sage, Geranium, Lemongrass, Neroli, Palmarosa, Rose, Sandalwood, Verbena, Ylang-Ylang.

MARS
Black Pepper, Cardamon, Clove, Coriander, Cumin, Ginger, Pine.

JUPITER
Hyssop, Marjoram, Nutmeg, Rosewood, Spikenard.

SATURN
Birch, Cajeput, Cedarwood, Celery, Eucalyptus, Juniper, Tea-Tree, Vetivert.

URANUS
Violet Leaf.

NEPTUNE
Seaweeds and mosses.

PLUTO
Cypress, Patchouli.

Blending with the Zodiac

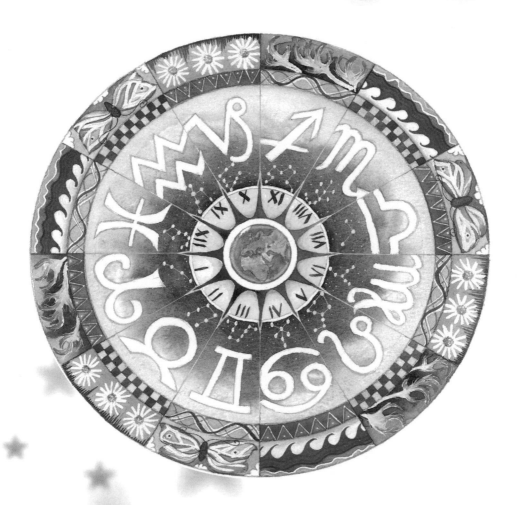

Blending with the Zodiac

Blending is one of the most fascinating facets of aromatherapy, one of the areas where art and science truly come together. We can approach blending from a therapeutic point of view, putting together several oils which each have certain properties that will be healing for the person we wish to help, or we can look at it from a purely aesthetic perspective and mix oils simply because they smell good together. In practice, though, the two go hand in hand: in making a therapeutic blend, we should not overlook the aroma of the end result. An unpleasant smell is far less likely to bring about the healing result we are looking for than something which is both therapeutically appropriate and enjoyable.

I recall a student once mixing Rose with Eucalyptus, for reasons that looked perfectly valid on paper, but she hadn't given any thought to what her blend would smell like. The overpowering aroma of the Eucalyptus completely cancelled the delicate Rose scent – a waste of costly Rose oil. The theoretical 'client' for whom this misalliance was intended was in need of some pampering and gentle nurture – hence the inclusion of Rose – but was hardly likely to have felt pampered when the only recognisable smell was the highly medicinal one of Eucalyptus. So, perhaps the first rule of blending should be 'Let your nose make the final decision'. If you are mixing essential oils for somebody else to use, whether as therapy or for fun, obviously they need to like it, too.

There are a number of other, more theoretical, rules involved in blending and if we then add astrological factors it might seem initially to make the whole business unduly complicated. Fortunately, though, the various approaches are not mutually exclusive and an astrological combination will often fulfil the criteria of more traditional systems of blending.

One system involves classifying aromas into different groups: woody, floral, herbal, spicy, oriental, etc. Most perfumes can be identified as belonging to one group or the other, but are made more interesting and balanced by the addition of very small amounts of perfuming materials from some of the other groups. Looking at the astrological parallels, you will find that the woody notes are mostly Saturn oils, many of the florals are Venus oils, and that Mercury has a high proportion of herbal plants among its oils. The spicy oils are mostly associated with Mars, while the oriental ones are mainly from plants of Jupiter or the Sun.

The best-known theory of blending, particularly in the world of perfumery, is that of Top, Middle and Bottom 'notes'. This was propounded by a 19th-century French perfumier, Piesse, who arranged perfuming ingredients (essential oils and others) on a stave, like a musical scale, according to their rate of evaporation. The top notes are those which evaporate fastest and the bottom (or base) notes those which do so very slowly, with the rest somewhere between the two extremes.

When you first sniff a complex perfume, the top note is what you notice immediately, but after a while you will pick up other elements as the top note evaporates and the middle and base notes become more prominent. This is why, when testing perfumes, it is never advisable to make an instant decision. Most aromatherapists bear the top/middle/bottom note theory in mind when mixing oils and virtually all commercial perfumes, and ready-made mixtures of essential oils, are formulated according to this system. In fact, from the Renaissance onwards, perfumiers had been combining elements in this way intuitively: what Piesse did was to formalise the system.

Towards the end of this chapter you will find a list of essential oils classified according to top, middle and bottom notes to help you create your own blends, though this is only a rough guide as there is as much disagreement over what constitutes a top note, a middle or a bottom one as there is about what oils can be attributed to which planet! This, I think, is largely due to the nature of essential oils themselves: many of them are very complex and contain top, middle and bottom notes within a single oil. Oil from identical plants can smell surprisingly different depending on where it was grown due to differences in soil and climate. Seasonal variations such as the weather during the growing and harvesting seasons can alter the character of an oil, too, sometimes sufficiently to change it from a top to a middle note or a middle to a base. The other reason for the lack of consensus is that the human nose is a wonderfully variable organ. All the same, the system is a sound one and a good starting point to work from.

Proportion is important: a top, middle and base note oil mixed in equal proportions is unlikely to produce a pleasing end result. One reason for this is that most of the base note oils are very powerful and could 'drown' whatever they were mixed with. A successful blend is most often composed of predominantly middle notes, with tiny additions of top and base notes. For example: Marguerite Maury, one of the pioneers of 20th-century aromatherapy, propounded a way of using essential oils in what she called the 'Individual Prescription' or 'Personal Perfume'. This was a blend of oils that was aesthetically pleasing at the same time as corresponding to her client's therapeutic needs and could be used by the aromatherapist in a massage oil and taken away by the client to use as a perfume on a day-to-day basis. For example, Madame S was in the habit of 'living in her head' and had been neglecting her body – she forgot to cook properly and would sit up late at night, absorbed in papers or books until she was exhausted – the perfume designed for her consisted of 98% Rose, with 1% Vetivert and 1% Black Pepper.

The end result 'works' whether you consider it as a perfume with a dusky, smoky undertone to the beautiful Rose aroma, or as a massage oil that will nurture Madame S's body (Rose), help her to be more grounded (Vetivert), and alleviate her fatigue (Black Pepper). It also corresponds to Piesse's system, with Black Pepper top note, Rose middle note and Vetivert base note. A mixture of equal parts of Rose, Black Pepper and Patchouli would not have been effective though: Patchouli is a very dominant aroma and would have overwhelmed the Rose just as the Eucalyptus did in the earlier example.

If we look at Madame S's birth data, we can see that the blend works equally well if we apply astrological principles. She has Sun in Aquarius, Libra rising and Aries Moon: the Vetivert will introduce the Earth element that is lacking, Rose (a Venus oil) will appeal to her Libran appreciation of beauty, while the Mars oil, Black Pepper, will give her the lift she needs and corresponds astrologically with her Moon.

So here you can see one way of using astrological data as a basis for designing blends. Taking the Sun, Moon and Ascendant in this way as a basis for selecting oils is, in my experience, a sound approach to astrological blending. It gives you the option of three oils which can be chosen for their therapeutic value or for their smell alone, and could easily include a top, middle and base note. If you plan to make a blend just for fun, as a bath mix, a room fragrance or perfume, you could customise the blend by taking three oils corresponding to the three signs, perhaps making the oil for the Sun sign the predominant one. If the blend is intended for therapeutic use you will need to consider the individual's needs, of course, as we did in the case of Madame S, and decide whether your blend is going to correspond to the elements that are represented by the three chart factors, or bring in an element or elements that are lacking. The oils discussed in the chapters on the individual signs and those attributed to their corresponding planets should give you plenty of ideas to work with and you will find some actual examples later in the chapter.

You might also consider whether the signature oils corresponding to a person's Sun, Moon and Ascendant would make a pleasing blend, preferably using the Sun sign's oil in the largest proportion. If the signature oils for their Sun and Ascendant would not mix well with that, even in tiny quantities, see what other oils appropriate for each sign could be used instead. The result will be a unique 'portrait in oils' of the person it was designed for.

If you are not sufficiently familiar with essential oils to decide which are top, middle or bottom notes (and remember, as we have already seen, there is very little agreement about this, anyway!), it is possible to draw analogies between the perfumier's scale of notes and the elements of Air, Fire, Water and Earth, with Air and Fire representing mostly top notes, Water ranging from top to middle, and Earth from middle to base.

We can see how this works in practice if we look at the plants attributed to each planet, and the element of the sign associated with that planet. For example, many of the oils attributed to airy Mercury/Gemini are top notes, though some, such as Fennel or Peppermint are unlikely to be aesthetically pleasing. Mars/Aries oils include such top notes as Black Pepper, while Citronella and Melissa, both Water/Moon oils, are valuable top notes, too. At the bottom end of the perfuming scale we have Saturn/ Capricorn oils such as Cedarwood, Juniper and Vetivert. Venus oils make an interesting study, ranging all the way from a top note in Lemongrass to a base note in Ylang-Ylang, but this makes perfect sense when we remember that Venus is associated with both earthy Taurus and airy Libra.

So far, we have only considered three chart factors and three corresponding oils, but if you have access to the full natal chart you could, in theory, play with many more. In reality, very complicated blends are seldom more successful than simple ones. (Commercial perfumiers do, in fact, combine many different ingredients but they are not dealing exclusively with essential oils and they are not concerned with the health and well-being of the people who use their products.) Blends of up to five oils can work very well both as perfumes and in treatments. From the therapeutic point of view, more than that can be counter-productive, bombarding the body with a confusing assortment of properties. It is usually possible to meet an individual's needs with three or four oils and, if not, I would suggest using two or three initially, in a massage for example, and introducing others as bath oils to be used later.

If you would like to experiment with blends based on a complete chart, try to pinpoint two other chart factors to add to the Sun, Moon and Ascendant. There may be an element that is poorly represented or completely absent, or empty signs or houses in the chart: you could pick an oil that brought in the missing element, or complemented an empty sign. There might be a planet in the sign where it is at its weakest, so you could include an oil related to that planet. The possibilities are endless and the more familiar you are with astrology, the more permutations you will be able to think of. For the less experienced, or the aromatherapist to whom this is all new, blends based on the Sun/Moon/Ascendant will serve very well.

But what if you don't have access to a person's birth data? Most people do know their Sun sign and, if not, you can identify it immediately by simply asking them the date of their birthday, and once you know that you could use their signature oil as a starting point. Most of the signature oils have a pleasing enough fragrance to stand as the main item in a blend, though you would need to be very sparing with some of the others to ensure they did not overwhelm any other oil mixed with them. Examples of the former are Rose (Taurus), Jasmine (Leo), Lavender (Virgo), Geranium or Palmarosa (Libra), Neroli (Aquarius) and Melissa (Pisces), while Vetivert (Capricorn) would be a good starting point for a masculine perfume. Only Rosemary (Aries), Basil (Gemini), Camomile (Cancer) and Patchouli (Scorpio) would need to be used in modest proportions.

How would you determine what oils to mix with the signature oil? One way would be to identify a complementary sign or planet. You might start by taking opposing pairs of signs in the birth chart: Aries opposite Libra gives us Rosemary and Geranium and in fact these two oils work very well in a blend: use more Geranium with a very little Rosemary for a woman's perfume, more Rosemary with a little Geranium for a man. Taurus/Scorpio gives us Rose and Patchouli: provided you use very, very little Patchouli it goes wonderfully well with Rose, as we saw in the example of Marguerite Maury's blend for Madame S. Gemini/Sagittarius would give us two spices, very compatible in cooking but not so nice for massage! Adding a little of Sagittarius's Black Pepper to an earthy oil such as Rosewood would be both grounding and energising for Gemini and, for a Sagittarian, would combine the fire element in the form of the spice with spiritual Jupiter: Rosewood. Cancer/Capricorn don't work terribly well either though, therapeutically, a very little Camomile with a larger proportion of Vetivert could well benefit either of these signs. To make an aesthetically pleasing perfume we need to look at other ways of making a blend for them such as choosing another Moon oil, perhaps Petitgrain or Melissa, either of which would go well with a smaller proportion of Vetivert. Leo/Aquarius would give us the most exquisite blend imaginable: Jasmine and Neroli. While Lavender and Melissa for Virgo and Pisces would work very well, too.

You can make all kinds of creative variations on this theme, by varying the proportions or substituting appropriate alternatives for one of the oils suggested.

In the next few pages you will find some suggestions for bath, massage and perfume blends for each of the 12 signs. The tonic/stimulant and relaxing blends are self-explanatory, but perhaps the restorative blends call for a little explanation: these are intended for those times when all of us need cossetting, whether we are physically a little below par, convalescent, a little bit depressed or sad, or simply in need of a little nurture. The ideal way to use them would be to receive a massage with the appropriate blend, but if that is not possible, a long, comfortably warm bath would be the next best solution. You could also try diffusing the blend as a room perfume or using it as a personal perfume. (In the latter cases, omit the vegetable oil.)

These are not hard-and-fast formulae but suggestions: for example, you can perfectly well use the bath blends for massage (but not always vice versa) and signs within the same element could try the blends designated for other signs in the same element.

★ BATH BLENDS

Each of the following blends makes a total of 6 drops, enough for one adult bath. For children between about five and 12 years, make up the 6 drops but use only half and keep the rest for another occasion. Most of the blends are unsuitable for infants and children under five: for them I suggest a drop or two of Camomile for Water signs, Lavender for Air signs, Mandarin for little Fiery ones, or Rose for Earth babies. If you know the child's Moon and/or Ascendant you could make gentle blends with any two of these oils – they all harmonise beautifully with each other. I would not recommend using more than two different oils at any one time for tiny children.

★ BATH BLENDS ★

Tonic/Stimulant	Relaxing	Restorative
ARIES		
Pine 3 drops	Lavender 3 drops	Rose 3 drops
Rosemary 2 drops	Petitgrain 2 drops	Mandarin 2 drops
Thyme 1 drop	Bergamot 1 drop	Geranium 1 drop
TAURUS		
Palmarosa 4 drops	Bergamot 4 drops	Rose 4 drops
Myrtle 1 drop	Ylang-Ylang 1 drop	Sandalwood 1 drop
Grapefruit 1 drop	Clary Sage 1 drop	Vetivert 1 drop
GEMINI		
Rosemary 3 drops	Lavender 4 drops	Benzoin 2 drops
Petitgrain 2 drops	Melissa 1 drop	Mandarin 3 drops
Basil 1 drop	Vetivert 1 drop	Basil 1 drop
CANCER		
Thyme 2 drops	Blue Camomile 2 drops	Rose 3 drops
Pine 2 drops	Lavender 2 drops	Bergamot 2 drops
Petitgrain 2 drops	Bergamot 2 drops	Elemi 1 drop
LEO		
Jasmine 4 drops	Clary Sage 3 drops	Jasmine 3 drops
Angelica Root 1 drop	Marjoram 2 drops	Mandarin 2 drops
Bay Laurel 1 drop	Lavender 1 drop	Elemi 1 drop
VIRGO		
Myrtle 3 drops	Lavender 4 drops	Rose 3 drops
Thyme 1 drop	Melissa 1 drop	Helichrysum 2 drops
Pine 2 drops	Mandarin 1 drop	Lavender 1 drop

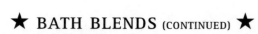

★ BATH BLENDS (CONTINUED) ★

Tonic/Stimulant	Relaxing	Restorative
LIBRA		
Pine 3 drops	Neroli 3 drops	Rose 3 drops
Manuka 2 drops	Bergamot 2 drops	Benzoin 2 drops
Grapefruit 1 drop	Lavender 1 drop	Orange 1 drop
SCORPIO		
Rosemary 3 drops	Clary Sage 3 drops	Bergamot 3 drops
Cypress 2 drops	Lavender 2 drops	Melissa 2 drops
Basil 1 drop	Blue Camomile 1 drop	Patchouli 1 drop
SAGITTARIUS		
Mandarin 4 drops	Clary Sage 3 drops	Rosewood 3 drops
Myrtle 1 drop	Rosewood 2 drops	Mandarin 2 drops
Pine 1 drop	Lavender 1 drop	Elemi 1 drop
CAPRICORN		
Cedarwood 4 drops	Marjoram 3 drops	Benzoin 3 drops
Manuka 1 drop	Lavender 2 drops	Mandarin 2 drops
Pine 1 drop	Clary Sage 1 drop	Vetivert 1 drop
AQUARIUS		
Pine 3 drops	Petitgrain 3 drops	Neroli 4 drops
Rosemary 2 drops	Lavender 2 drops	Rose 1 drop
Lime 1 drop	Bergamot 1 drop	Ylang-Ylang 1 drop
PISCES		
Cedarwood 4 drops	Lavender 3 drops	Ylang-Ylang 3 drops
Verbena 1 drop	Petitgrain 2 drops	Geranium 2 drops
Pine 1 drop	Ylang-Ylang 1 drop	Melissa 1 drop

★ MASSAGE BLENDS

Each of the massage blends totals 18 drops of essential oil, to be added to 30 ml of carrier oil. This is sufficient for a full-body massage. If you want to use the same blend more than once, use multiples of 30 ml and store in a brown or other opaque bottle. Don't make up too much at a time, though, as the carrier oils do not keep as long as essential oils. You will see that in some instances the suggested massage blend is the same as the bath blend for the same sign and purpose, though the proportions may differ: this reflects the fact that all the components are safe to use in a bath. To make a massage oil for a baby or very young child, stay with the recommendations for bath oils, using Camomile, Lavender, Mandarin or Rose. Add 3 drops to 10 ml of carrier oil – this is quite enough for a baby massage.

★ MASSAGE BLENDS ★

Tonic/Stimulant	Relaxing	Restorative
ARIES		
Pine 12 drops	Lavender 9 drops	Rose 5 drops
Rosemary 5 drops	Petitgrain 6 drops	Orange 12 drops
Black Pepper 1 drop	Grapefruit 3 drops	Nutmeg 1 drop
In 30 ml Sunflower oil		
TAURUS		
Orange 12 drops	Bergamot 12 drops	Rose 12 drops
Lemongrass 4 drops	Ylang-Ylang 3 drops	Sandalwood 3 drops
Nutmeg 2 drops	Clary Sage 3 drops	Helichrysum 3 drops
In 30 ml Almond oil		
GEMINI		
Rosemary 8 drops	Lavender 10 drops	Mandarin 10 drops
Orange 6 drops	Melissa 6 drops	Helichrysum 6 drops
Basil 4 drops	Vetivert 2 drops	Nutmeg 2 drops
In 30 ml Grapeseed oil		

235

★ MASSAGE BLENDS (CONTINUED)

Tonic/Stimulant	Relaxing	Restorative
CANCER		
Lemon 8 drops	Blue Camomile 10 drops	Bergamot 12 drops
Thyme 8 drops	Lavender 6 drops	Frankincense 3 drops
Ginger 2 drops	Melissa 2 drops	Blue Camomile 3 drops
In 30 ml Sesame oil		
LEO		
Jasmine 10 drops	Clary Sage 10 drops	Jasmine 10 drops
Angelica 6 drops	Marjoram 6 drops	Neroli 7 drops
Ginger 2 drops	Lavender 2 drops	Nutmeg 1 drop
In 30 ml Sunflower oil		
VIRGO		
Myrtle 10 drops	Lavender 10 drops	Rose 15 drops
Grapefruit 6 drops	Melissa 4 drops	Neroli 2 drops
Thyme 2 drops	Petitgrain 4 drops	Lavender 1 drop
In 30 ml Almond oil		
LIBRA		
Pine 9 drops	Neroli 9 drops	Rose 9 drops
Manuka 6 drops	Bergamot 6 drops	Benzoin 6 drops
Grapefruit 3 drop	Lavender 3 drop	Orange 3 drop
In 30 ml Grapeseed oil		
SCORPIO		
Cypress 12 drops	Clary Sage 9 drops	Bergamot 10 drops
Rosemary 5 drops	Lavender 6 drops	Orange 6 drops
Basil 1 drop	Melissa 3 drops	Patchouli 2 drops
In 30 ml Sesame oil		
SAGITTARIUS		
Myrtle 8 drops	Rosewood 9 drops	Rosewood 10 drops
Orange 8 drops	Clary Sage 6 drops	Orange 5 drops
Black Pepper 2 drops	Lavender 3 drops	Frankincense 3 drops
In 30 ml Sunflower oil		

★ MASSAGE BLENDS (CONTINUED) ★

Tonic/Stimulant	Relaxing	Restorative
CAPRICORN		
Cedarwood 10 drops	Marjoram 10 drops	Orange 10 drops
Manuka 6 drops	Lavender 4 drops	Benzoin 6 drops
Ginger 2 drops	Clary Sage 4 drops	Vetivert 2 drops
In 30 ml Almond oil		
AQUARIUS		
Pine 10 drops	Petitgrain 9 drops	Neroli 12 drops
Lime 5 drops	Lavender 6 drops	Rose 3 drops
Nutmeg 3 drops	Bergamot 3 drops	Ylang-Ylang 3 drops
In 30 ml Grapeseed oil		
PISCES		
Cedarwood 12 drops	Melissa 9 drops	Melissa 9 drops
Verbena 3 drops	Lavender 6 drops	Geranium 6 drops
Pine 3 drops	Ylang-Ylang 3 drops	Ylang-Ylang 3 drops
In 30 ml Sesame oil		

★ PERFUME BLENDS

The perfume formulae adhere a little less strictly to astrological principles than the bath and massage blends. This is because the aesthetic appeal of the finished aroma is even more important in this context than in therapeutic blends, not that the latter should ever be unpleasant. A 'perfume' (or aftershave, cologne, body-splash, etc.) must, by definition, smell pleasing, so all the strongly 'medicinal-smelling' oils have to be ruled out (remember the Rose and Eucalyptus disaster I wrote about earlier). You will see that certain oils recur frequently: many of these have been used as perfume ingredients for well over a thousand years and it is no coincidence that the majority of them are oils associated with Venus, with the connotation of luxury, aesthetic and sensuous pleasure. Despite that, we can still create an astrological balance in the blends by introducing oils from other planets, sometimes in very small proportions.

237

As I wrote in the early part of this chapter, "Let your nose make the final decision" though the final decisions on the blends that follow were made not by my nose, but by the noses of the many volunteers who tested the blends appropriate to their own Sun sign. They sampled the perfumes and commented on them; if they were not entirely happy I modified the blend until they were, sometimes by changing the proportion of the various oils, sometimes by replacing one or more of them. Your nose, or the noses of people for whom you would like to make perfume, may not like the end results as much as my volunteers did, so please feel free to adapt the formulae in the same way. Experiment with different proportions, and if you want to substitute an oil it is always possible to find one that is either associated with the same planet or at least the same element, so that the astrological basis of the blend is not compromised.

Aroma preferences are highly individual. They are influenced by such diverse factors as minuscule physiological differences between one person's nose and the next, – memories pleasant or unpleasant associated with smells, diet, cultural conditioning – even skin and hair colour, as aromas can smell differently on the skin of a blonde from that of a redhead, and different again on a brunette.

If we consider them from an astrological point of view they may be influenced as much by the Ascendant as by the Sun sign, so it could be interesting to try the blends corresponding to your Ascendant (the bath and massage ones, as well as the perfume). The Moon in a chart might be another influence, so look at blends for your Moon's sign. A third possibility is where there is a concentration of planets in one sign: that sign will have a correspondingly strong influence.

Each of these perfume blends totals 5 ml of essential oil. To make a perfume such as you might buy commercially, this would need to be added to perfume-grade alcohol but, in the United Kingdom, it is not possible to buy this without a licence (which is difficult to obtain). There are some alternatives to alcohol which can be obtained from specialist aromatherapy suppliers, but essential-oil blends can also be used directly on the skin as a perfume without dilution. Be very sparing with them, using only a drop or two at a time. For anybody with sensitive skin, test a single drop first.

If you live outside the UK and can obtain perfume-grade alcohol, mix the 5 ml essential-oil blend with 20 to 25 ml alcohol to make a full-strength perfume, with 50 ml to make an eau de parfum, or with 100 ml to make an eau de toilette. Perfume blends benefit by being left to mature for a few weeks before use, especially if you are able to use an alcohol base. If you are in a hurry, try at least to leave the blend for a few hours before using it, to allow the different aromas to fully integrate with each other.

★ PERFUME BLENDS ★

For an Aries Man

Grapefruit 60 drops

Bergamot 25 drops

Rosemary 8 drops

Bay Laurel 6 drops

Black Pepper 1 drop

For a Taurus Man

Sandalwood 46 drops

Rose 40 drops

Helichrysum 10 drops

Coriander 3 drops

Patchouli 1 drop

For a Gemini Man

Grapefruit 55 drops

Bay Laurel 30 drops

Myrtle 8 drops

Angelica Root 5 drops

Basil 2 drops

For an Aries Woman

Bergamot 55 drops

Rose 30 drops

Geranium 10 drops

Black Pepper 3 drops

Ginger 2 drops

For a Taurus Woman

Rose 60 drops

Sandalwood 18 drops

Helichrysum 18 drops

Ginger 3 drops

Patchouli 1 drop

For a Gemini Woman

Mimosa 70 drops

Mandarin 10 drops

Helichrysum 10 drops

Angelica Root 9 drops

Basil 1 drop

For a Cancer Man

Cypress 45 drops

Melissa 25 drops

Grapefruit 20 drops

Blue Camomile 5 drops

Vetivert 5 drops

For a Leo Man

Jasmine 50 drops

Neroli 30 drops

Cedarwood 10 drops

Bay Laurel 8 drops

Black Pepper 2 drops

For a Virgo Man

Petitgrain 70 drops

Neroli 10 drops

Lavender 10 drops

Cedarwood 7 drops

Myrtle 3 drops

For a Libra Man

Sandalwood 45 drops

Rose 42 drops

Lemongrass 8 drops

Cardamon 3 drops

Angelica Root 2 drops

For a Scorpio Man

Melissa 40 drops

Cypress 35 drops

Patchouli 10 drops

Lemongrass 10 drops

Ginger 5 drops

For a Cancer Woman

Rose 35 drops

Melissa 30 drops

Ylang-Ylang 20 drops

Blue Camomile 10 drops

Vetivert 5 drops

For a Leo Woman

Neroli 50 drops

Rose 30 drops

Petitgrain 10 drops

Vetivert 8 drops

Green Pepper 2 drops

For a Virgo Woman

Rose 70 drops

Neroli 10 drops

Lavender 10 drops

Petitgrain 8 drops

Cedarwood 2 drops

For a Libra Woman

Rose 80 drops

Geranium 10 drops

Sandalwood 5 drops

Violet Leaf 3 drops

Angelica Root 2 drops

For a Scorpio Woman

Melissa 50 drops

Lemongrass 20 drops

Cypress 15 drops

Patchouli 10 drops

Ginger 5 drops

For a Sagittarius Man

Rosewood 55 drops

Palmarosa 25 drops

Benzoin 10 drops

Nutmeg 5 drops

Black Pepper 5 drops

For a Capricorn Man

Vetivert 40 drops

Sandalwood 40 drops

Juniper 10 drops

Lime 5 drops

Cedarwood 5 drops

For an Aquarius Man

Petitgrain 40 drops

Lime 30 drops

Neroli 15 drops

Violet Leaf 10 drops

Pine 5 drops

For a Pisces Man

Melissa 30 drops

Lime 25 drops

Cypress 25 drops

Geranium 15 drops

Ylang-Ylang 5 drops

For a Sagittarius Woman

Rosewood 45 drops

Rose 30 drops

Benzoin 10 drops

Spikenard 10 drops

Black Pepper 5 drops

For a Capricorn Woman

Orange 36 drops

Sandalwood 32 drops

Vetivert 24 drops

Juniper 4 drops

Lime 4 drops

For an Aquarius Woman

Neroli 50 drops

Violet Leaf 20 drops

Bergamot 10 drops

Mimosa 10 drops

Ylang-Ylang 10 drops

For a Pisces Woman

Melissa 35 drops

Lime 20 drops

Geranium 20 drops

Cypress 15 drops

Ylang-Ylang 10 drops

I hope this chapter will be a starting point for your creative experiments in making your own astrologically based blends. As long as you observe the safety factors, such as avoiding spices and some of the citrus oils in bath blends*, not exceeding 6 drops for a bath, using 3 drops of essential oil to 5 ml of carrier oil for massage (3 drops to 10 ml or even

*Note: Most of the spices and some of the citrus oils are safe to use on the skin when diluted in a carrier oil but can cause uncomfortable stinging if used in the bath.

15 ml for infants), the field is wide open for you to experiment. The sky is, quite literally, the limit: your perfume palette includes all the signs, all the planets and all the corresponding essential oils. Enjoy them!

★ ESSENTIAL OILS CLASSIFIED BY TOP, MIDDLE AND BOTTOM NOTES

TOP NOTES

Basil, Bergamot, Black Pepper, Cajeput, Caraway, Citronella, Eucalyptus, Lemon, Lemongrass, Melissa, Myrtle, Palmarosa, Parsley, Peppermint, Rosemary, Thyme, Verbena.

MIDDLE NOTES

Camomile, Cardamon, Carrot, Clary Sage, Coriander, Cumin, Cypress, Fennel, Geranium, Helichrysum, Hyssop, Juniper, Lavender, Mandarin, Marjoram, Mimosa, Neroli, Nutmeg, Petitgrain, Pine, Orange, Rose, Violet Leaf.

BOTTOM NOTES

Angelica, Benzoin, Cedarwood, Clove, Elemi, Frankincense, Ginger, Jasmine, Myrrh, Patchouli, Rosewood, Sandalwood, Spikenard, Vetivert, Ylang-Ylang.

Putting it all together

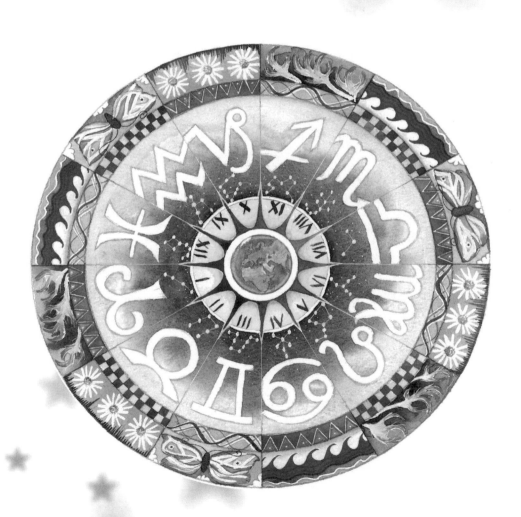

Putting it all together

A SAMPLE BIRTH CHART AND AROMATHERAPY TREATMENT

To help put all these different factors together, and to see how they might help in deciding on aromatherapy treatment, it is time to look at a sample birth chart, and the health problems experienced by the person whose chart this is. Let's call him Charles. He is happy to have his chart used in this way but it would, of course, be unethical to disclose his identity.

At the time of consulting, his physical problems included sinusitis leading to frequent, severe headaches and muscular pain in the neck and shoulders. He was also exhausted after a lengthy overseas teaching tour and said he felt a bit depressed because he had put on weight, partly through staying in hotels, eating out and being offered much hospitality during the tour. He was very willing to give me all his birth data – time and place as well as date – and welcomed the fact that I would draw on astrology in planning his treatment. He had had a natal chart drawn up some time previously and, although he had forgotten his ascendant, he knew both his Sun and Moon signs, so I was able to incorporate that information straight away, without needing to wait until I could calculate a chart.

My first choice of oil was Rosemary, the signature oil for Aries, to restore some of his energy and at the same time help clear his sinuses and relieve the headaches. I blended this with Bergamot, to lift the depression, and Juniper, which is detoxifying, in a 3:2:1 ratio. All three of these are Sun oils which would bring comforting warmth to both body and spirit, and I mixed them into sunflower oil for good measure.

At this first visit I gave Charles a face, head and neck massage, including some drainage strokes on the face to help clear his sinuses. His face was tender and painful in places so this had to be done very gently. I spent a lot of time easing tight muscles in his neck and shoulders, not only to reduce the pain he felt in that area but also because tight neck muscles can restrict blood supply to the brain and this, as well as the sinusitis, could be contributing to his headaches. I did not talk about food at this first visit, either in relation to his sinusitis or weight increase, because he was already beating himself up about it and was tired and in pain. These are not the best circumstances in which to offer dietary advice! I decided to return to this at a later date...always assuming that Charles would come back for further treatment. For home use I recommended steam inhalations with Rosemary each morning and with Lavender at night. This should help to clear his sinuses, give him a little energy boost in the mornings and promote good, restorative sleep at night. He did, in fact, make an appointment for a second visit and I calculated a chart for him in readiness, so by the time of this second appointment I was aware of his Leo Ascendant and all the other factors shown by his chart.

Let's look at this chart, and then consider what it might tell us about Charles' physical and emotional strengths and weaknesses and how that knowledge could be applied to his aromatherapy treatment.

In chart interpretation we always look first at the general shape of the chart, then at the Sun, Ascendant and Moon, then the other planets. The overall shape of the chart shows a marked emphasis on the latter houses, with only two planets in the personal houses, suggesting a life lived more in public than in private, possibly at some cost to personal happiness. You can also see that there are no planets in his seventh House of Partnerships, and that this house has Aquarius on the cusp which may possibly imply an unconventional attitude to relationships or somebody who is a bit of a loner.

Charles has Sun in Aries, which tells us that he is likely to be a dynamic, energetic person, possibly a pioneer of some kind, with qualities of leadership. It also alerts us to the fact that he may experience physical problems associated with the head, particularly headaches, sinusitis, earache, etc., and that there is some danger of burn-out as Ariens will often push themselves to their physical limits, and beyond.

He has Leo on the Ascendant: quite compatible with an Aries Sun, as these are both Fire signs. Leo likes to be in the limelight, to be the centre of attention, and as a personality trait this can integrate easily with the leadership role the Aries Sun suggests and the emphasis on the 'public' areas of his chart. Leo has an affinity with the heart and lungs so we should be on the lookout for any signs of disease affecting these organs.

His Moon is in Taurus, a good, solid Earth sign which will help to modify some of the excesses implied by Sun and Ascendant both in Fire

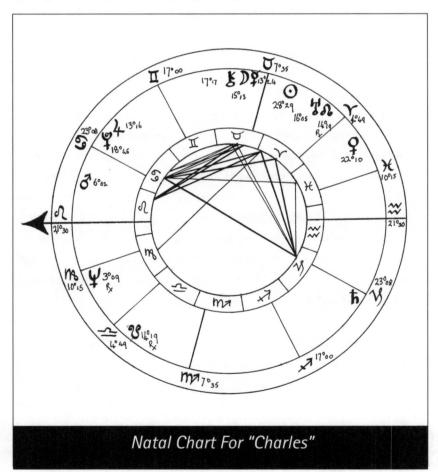

Natal Chart For "Charles"

signs, but may lead to different excesses in the form of overindulgence in food, wine, etc. Taurus has an affinity with the neck and shoulders, so we should also look out for problems that affect those areas: sore throats, laryngitis, muscular pain in this area, etc. Charles has Chiron conjunct his Moon and when we see Chiron this close to a planet it is often an indication that healing is needed around issues associated with that planet. In the case of the Moon, these might be issues to do with nurture or mothering and in Taurus this could manifest as problems around food.

Charles has Neptune in the first house: he might well be a highly spiritual person, very sensitive but conversely he could have an addictive personality. The fact that Neptune is Trine to his Sun in the ninth house (the house of Philosophy, Higher Learning, etc.) makes it much more likely that the former is true. In fact, we see a very big emphasis on the ninth house, with two planets in that house, plus his North Node so he is very likely to be drawn to spiritual, religious or philosophical exploration. With Uranus as one of those planets his explorations may be of an unconventional nature.

His Mercury is only a fraction of a degree away from his Midheaven, the 10th house cusp, and conjunct his Moon and Chiron just inside the 10th house. With the planet of communication right on the M.C. (Midheaven) like this we can expect this person's role in the world to involve communication, and with the Moon and Chiron also in the 10th house it is likely that the communication will be something to do with nurturing, health and healing. These three planets and the M.C. are all in Taurus, giving a good, solid grounding to his career, which is helped and given structure by Trines to the Moon and Chiron from Saturn in Capricorn.

How does this translate into real life? How does it affect his health and the decisions we might take about aromatherapy treatments?

Well, Charles is indeed a leader and pioneer: he was involved with complementary medicine before it was widely popular and teaches in several continents. He is a charismatic speaker, bringing a spiritual approach to his healing practice, and has written a number of books and magazine articles.

I'm sure you can see, too, how the symptoms he described at his first visit relate to what we see in his chart. His Sun sign, Aries, is associated with the head: sinusitis and headaches being common problems for this sign. Taurus, where his Moon is situated, is linked to the neck and shoulders where he was experiencing pain and stiffness. Many Taureans have a tendency to overindulge in good food, wine, etc., and with the Moon in this sign, rather than the Sun or Ascendant, it is likely that such indulgences are linked to the emotions as much as, or more than, to simple enjoyment of the good things of life. In this instance, the conjunction between Charles' Moon and Chiron hinted that this was even more likely to be true.

Looking at the Leo ascendant, we remember that Leo is associated with the heart and although Charles has no history of heart disease he would be well advised to watch his food intake and exercise regime, so I resolved to tackle this topic. Because of Leo's tendency towards depression, I wondered whether his admission of being "a bit" depressed was an understatement, though I would not voice my suspicion unless Charles touched on this topic himself. I made a mental note, too, that he has Capricorn on the cusp of the sixth house which might (through its association with Saturn) also suggest depression. A Capricorn sixth house can also denote rigidity in the body, so I decided to watch the stiffness he complained of in his neck and shoulders to see whether it persisted.

At the second visit he reported that he had had no more headaches since I first saw him, his face was less tender though his nose was still "stuffy" as he put it. He felt less exhausted, but still had less energy than he would like. As the first oils I had chosen seemed to be doing exactly what I hoped, I used the same blend for a full-body massage, but changed the ratio to equal parts of each oil. He had slightly less need of the stimulant action of Rosemary, and a little more

Juniper would help clear his body of the toxins that were still causing catarrh.

While he was resting after his massage, I asked him if he felt more in control of what he was eating, now that he was not dependent on hotel catering or his hosts' hospitality. He admitted, rather ruefully, that he did not. He said he was often too tired or too busy to cook properly for himself and would often bring in takeaway food or oven-ready meals or just snack, also that he tended to eat for comfort when he was unhappy.

"And you're unhappy at present?" I asked. He nodded and was silent for a moment, then began to tell me that his marriage had ended in divorce some years previously, and a new relationship which he hoped would be long-term had foundered. He thought that some of his tiredness stemmed from the effort of hiding his depression from his regular clients and the groups he had been teaching. On top of this, he felt embarrassed and even ashamed that he couldn't heal his own emotional problems. "Physician, heal thyself!" he said in an ironic tone.

We may extend the link between Leo and the heart to the metaphorical 'heart', to his depression and the fact that this seems to be related to relationships. Leos can become trapped in terrible depressions, of long duration, from which they see no way out. Jasmine is one of the most wonderful oils for long-term depression and, of course, it is the signature oil for his Leo Ascendant so I suggested that he used Jasmine at home in baths and as a room-fragrancer if he enjoyed it.

At the third visit I changed the emphasis and switched to Jasmine blended with a very little Black Pepper (Mars) for his massage, giving him a tonic/cleansing blend of Rosemary with Cypress for bathing. By this time I had established that he bathed more often in the morning than at night, so Rosemary was appropriate. Cypress is associated with Saturn, therefore stability, and I could see that travelling in connection with his work mitigated against a steady routine and stable home life. I had noted the empty fourth house, which alerted me to this possibility, and our conversation about his failed relationship confirmed that he lived alone when, indeed, he was at home. I got the impression that 'home' for Charles at that time was little more than a base from which to take off on his travels.

Charles continued to see me for treatment at roughly weekly intervals, sometimes longer when his teaching schedule intervened. He became more relaxed in my presence so I was able to talk with him, first, about catarrh-forming foods such as wheat and dairy products and, later, to suggest that counselling might be one way to resolve his depression. He admitted that he was very reluctant to see a counsellor because of his high-profile involvement in healing and teaching.

So I told him the story of Chiron, the Wounded Healer, and he understood the metaphor immediately. The position of Chiron in the 'career' area of Charles' chart is so very symbolic in this respect: he *is* a wounded healer.

He promised to think again about counselling: in the meantime I suggested that he might try taking St John's Wort (another Sun herb) as well as continuing to use a variety of antidepressant essential oils to lift the dark moods when they hit him.

My professional involvement with Charles ended soon after this session, as I moved to the other side of the country. From time to time he sends me postcards from different parts of the world, once a long letter to let me know he had eventually followed my advice about counselling and was glad that he had. Remembering which year he was born, I realised that he had eventually decided to seek counselling when he was 51, that is to say, in the year of his Chiron Return, which is so often a major turning point in our healing journey.

Perhaps I should end this chapter by saying that, as an experienced aromatherapist, I may well have chosen the same oils and much the same programme of treatment without the help of astrology. Having Charles' natal chart to hand certainly confirmed my intuitive choice of oils and probably led me to look at certain areas of his life sooner than I might otherwise have done and before he spoke of them himself. I chose his chart and case history to use as an example here because they demonstrate so clearly the links between signs, parts of the body, the sort of problems that might be expected, and how looking at the planetary affinities of plants can help to resolve them.

I have certainly found the input from astrology almost like a 'second opinion' when dealing with cases more complex and puzzling than Charles'. It has been especially valuable when dealing with people who are reluctant to talk about themselves, their lives and their problems or who perhaps do not make a connection between the immediate problem for which they are seeking help and other areas of their experience. Charles was a very self-aware and articulate person but, clearly, not everyone who looks to us for help via aromatherapy will have the same level of clarity.

In almost every instance, a birth-chart analysis has helped me to understand facets of a person's character faster than I would have done through the usual means of talking with them (though of course a chart can never replace the value of talking) and helped me to select the most appropriate oils, blends and methods of application sooner than I might have done without that input.

If you are perhaps fairly new to the profession of aromatherapy, or a non-professional using oils to help yourself, your family or friends, the guidance you can get from a natal chart, or even just somebody's Sun sign, may be even more welcome. If you are a seasoned aromatherapist you may still find new depths of understanding by considering the astrological background of your clients.

May I suggest some exercises to help you get into the habit of working in this way?

First, study your OWN natal chart! (Or just consider your Sun sign if you do not have a chart available.) You know yourself better than you know anybody else; you know what your own problems are, physical or emotional, major or minor, and when they began; you know about the major events in your life and when they took place. See how much of this you can relate to the chart in terms of signs, planets, houses, and so forth.

Then look at the affinities between plants and planets, plants and signs and, especially, your signature oil and see if you can make a treatment plan for yourself. If you have any ongoing problems, you could try this out in practice. If not, you can work out what you might have done in relation to past problems or illnesses.

Next, take the the charts of two or three people you know well – family or close friends – and repeat the process. If you don't already know about their past problems, ask them for feedback about the accuracy of your findings. If they are willing to try any oils you suggest for current problems, so much the better – you can test the efficiency of your theories.

Then try to get some charts, or any astrological data you can find, for people you don't know so well and repeat the process. Newspapers and magazines often carry details of celebrities' birthdays – see if you can guess, on the basis of their Sun sign, what their physical strengths and weaknesses are, and decide what oils you would choose if you were called on to help them. Some astrology magazines and books print charts or birth data for well known people, both past and present, and with these you could repeat the exercise basing your decisions on a complete chart.

Only by studying charts and relating them to real people will you learn to put all this theory into practice. The more you do this, the easier it will become, until it is second nature.

Astrological
Aromatherapy

Where do we go from here?

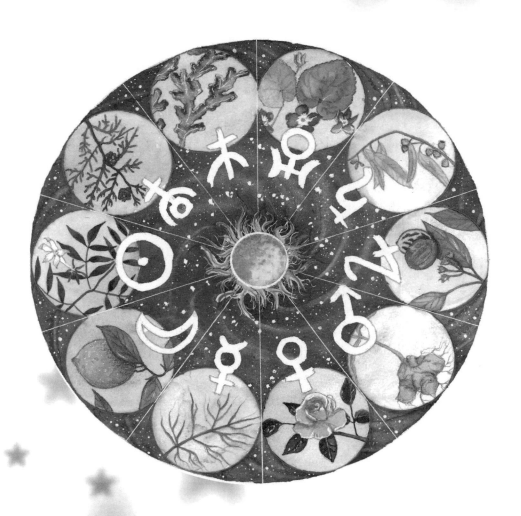

Where do we go from here?

If you have stayed with me this far, I hope that some of my enthusiasm for combining the two ancient arts of aromatherapy and astrology will have communicated itself to you, and that you will want to continue experimenting in this field. So, what are the next steps?

I would suggest that you start modestly with whichever of the two disciplines is least familiar to you. If you are knowledgeable about essential oils, start by working with oils and Sun signs, then try to incorporate the Moon and Ascendant before you attempt to relate the oils to a complete natal chart. You will find a number of books listed in the Appendix which will expand on what you have read here, and there are any number of reputable astrology courses available, from those for beginners right through to diploma courses for people who want to practise as astrological counsellors. Some local authorities offer classes at their adult education institutes, and in many towns you will find locally based astrologers offering talks and classes privately. All the astrological organisations listed in the Appendix offer training courses, lectures, seminars, and in some cases residential summer schools.

If you think you will want to draw on astrology regularly as an adjunct to aromatherapy treatment, you would probably find some appropriate software useful. With the help of a computer it is possible to draw up an accurate natal chart or investigate a person's current transits in minutes rather than the several hours that it would take to do the same work manually. Do beware, though, of computer 'interpretations'. Even the best of them can only be an approximation.

Conversely, if you are an experienced astrologer, don't rush out and buy a huge selection of essential oils. Try a selection of, perhaps, six oils and work with them until you are thoroughly familiar with their properties before adding new oils to your collection one at a time. My remarks about reading and training courses in astrology apply equally well to aromatherapy. You will find some suggestions for further reading listed at the end of this book and there are local authority courses almost everywhere, as well as many other courses ranging from weekends, for people who want to use a few oils at home, to full-scale certificated courses leading to professional qualifications. The governing bodies listed in the Appendix will provide lists of accredited schools.

You may want to go far more deeply into the connection between astrology and healing by studying formal medical astrology, or look into the close relationship between vedic astrology and ayurvedic medicine. The connection between signs, planets and the chakras is another fascinating area of study.

I beg you, whatever your previous experience or training, to look at the sky. The stars and planets are far more than mere symbols: they are *real* and there in space for us to wonder at. If you are not already familiar with them, a number of national newspapers feature a weekly or monthly 'sky at night' column which will show you where to look for particular constellations and planets at different times of the year, or you may like to get a calendar with a star map for each month. The Moon is our closest neighbour in space and is easy to observe in all her phases: try to notice how you feel, how the people around you behave and how that reflects the different energies which prevail at each phase.

Just as the planets are more than abstract symbols, aromatics are more than liquids in little brown bottles, so look at aromatic plants, too, and if you have a garden or even a windowsill, try to grow as many as you can and observe their colours, their shapes and their habit of growth. Smell them, taste them, touch them; it will heighten your understanding of essential oils more than anything else I know.

Finally, I wish you the greatest delight on your journey of discovery.

★ GLOSSARY OF AROMATHERAPY TERMS

ABSOLUTE	Material obtained from flowers by enfleurage (q.v.) or solvent extraction.
ANALGESIC	Reduces pain.
ANAPHRODISIAC	Reduces sexual response.
ANTIBIOTIC	Combats infection within the body.
ANTIDEPRESSANT	Helps to lift the mood.
ANTIFUNGAL	Combats fungal infections.
ANTI-INFLAMMATORY	Reduces inflammation.
ANTISEPTIC	Prevents or combats bacterial infection locally.
ANTISPASMODIC	Prevents or relieves muscular spasms.
ANTIVIRAL	Kills or inhibits the growth of viruses.
APHRODISIAC	Increases sexual response.
ASTRINGENT	Tightens the tissues, reduces fluid loss.
BACTERICIDE	Kills bacteria.
BECHIC	Relieves coughs.
CARRIER OIL	An unperfumed vegetable oil with which essential oils are diluted for massage and other applications.
CEPHALIC	Stimulates mental activity.
CYTOPHYLACTIC	A cell regenerator.
DEODORANT	Reduces or prevents odour.
DETOXIFYING	Helps clear the body of impurities.
DIURETIC	Increases production of urine.
EMMENAGOGUE	Encourages menstruation.
ENFLEURAGE	A method of extraction in which flower petals are laid on muslin soaked in oil or fat until the essence has been absorbed.

ESSENTIAL OIL	A highly concentrated, volatile compound extracted from plants by means of distillation. The basic material of aromatherapy.
EXPECTORANT	Helps expel phlegm.
FEBRIFUGE	Reduces fever.
FLORAL OIL	See INFUSED OIL.
FUNGICIDAL	Kills or inhibits the growth of yeasts, moulds, etc.
HEPATIC	Strengthens the liver.
HERBAL EXTRACT	A water-based extract from a medicinal plant.
HERBAL OIL	See INFUSED OIL.
HYDROLAT	The water which is collected when plants have been distilled to extract the essential oil. Hydrolats contain many extracts from the plant.
HYDROSOL	See HYDROLAT.
HYPERTENSIVE	Raises blood pressure.
HYPOTENSIVE	Reduces blood pressure.
IMMUNO-STIMULANT	Strengthens the body's defences against infection.
INFUSED OIL	A vegetable oil in which plant material (leaves or petals) have been steeped until their active principles have been absorbed.
MUCOLYTIC	Breaks down catarrh.
NERVINE	Strengthens the nervous system.
RUBEFACIENT	Produces warmth and redness when applied to the skin.
SEDATIVE	Calms the nervous system.

STIMULANT	Increases activity of a specific organ or the whole body.
TINCTURE	An extract obtained by soaking plant material in alcohol.
TONIC	Strengthens the whole body or a specific organ.
UTERINE	Has a tonic action on the womb.
VASOCONSTRICTOR	Causes small blood vessels to contract.
VASODILATOR	Causes small blood vessels to expand.
VULNERARY	Helps wounds to heal.

★ GLOSSARY OF ASTROLOGICAL TERMS

ANGLE	One of four sensitive points on a natal chart (see ASCENDANT, DESCENDANT, I.C. and M.C.).
ARIES	The Ram, first sign of the Zodiac.
ASCENDANT	The point on a natal chart that shows which sign was rising on the Eastern horizon at the moment of birth. Marks the start of the first house.
ASPECT	The spatial relationship between two planets, or between a planet and an Angle (see CONJUNCTION, OPPOSITION, SEXTILE, SQUARE and TRINE).
AQUARIUS	The Water-carrier, the 11th sign of the Zodiac.
CANCER	The Crab. The fourth sign of the Zodiac.
CAPRICORN	The Goat. The 10th sign of the Zodiac.
CARDINAL	One of the three Qualities of the signs. Cardinal Signs are initiators, inquisitive and active.

CHIRON	A large asteroid orbiting between Saturn and Uranus. In mythology, Chiron was a centaur known as the Wounded Healer.
CONJUNCTION	Two planets at the same degree in a chart, or very nearly so.
CUSP	The division between one sign and the next, or one house and the next in a chart. Usually refers to the beginning of a sign or house.
DESCENDANT	The point on a natal chart that shows which sign was setting on the Western horizon at the moment of birth. Marks the start of the seventh house.
ECLIPTIC	The Sun's *apparent* path through the Zodiac.
ELEMENT	Each sign is attributed to one of the four elements: Fire, Earth, Air and Water which describes something about the nature of that sign.
EPHEMERIS	A table showing the daily positions of the Sun, Moon and planets.
FIXED	One of the three Qualities of the signs. Fixed signs are stable, reliable and dislike change.
GEMINI	The Twins. The third sign of the Zodiac.
GRAND TRINE	A pattern seen in some natal charts where three planets all form a Trine to each other.

HOUSE	A division of the natal chart indicating different areas of life experience.
HOUSE SYSTEM	One of several methods of calculating the position of the houses, the best-known being Equal House, Koch and Placidus.
I.C. or IMUM COELI	The "Lowest heaven", i.e. the lowest point on a chart, it relates to our home and experience of family. In most house systems marks the start of the fourth house.
JUPITER	The fifth planet from the Sun. Chief of all the gods of Olympus in classical mythology.
LEO	The Lion. The fifth sign of the Zodiac.
LIBRA	The Scales. The seventh sign of the Zodiac.
LIGHTS	The Sun and Moon in astrology.
MARS	The fourth planet from the Sun. God of war in classical mythology.
M.C. or MIDHEAVEN	The highest point on the chart, it relates to our career or position in the world, and usually marks the beginning of the 10th house.
MERCURY	The nearest planet to the Sun. The Messenger of the Gods in classical mythology.

MUTABLE	One of the three Qualities of signs. Mutable signs are flexible, adaptable and ready to change.
NEPTUNE	The eighth planet from the Sun. God of the Sea in classical mythology.
NODES	Points where the Moon's path crosses the Ecliptic.
OPPOSITION	An aspect in which two planets are directly opposite each other, 180° apart on the circle. Regarded as a 'hard' aspect, it demands that we pay attention to the issues it indicates.
PISCES	The Fishes. The 12th sign of the Zodiac.
PLANET	One of the planets of the solar system, namely Mercury, Venus, Mars, (Earth), Jupiter, Saturn, Uranus, Neptune and Pluto in order of distance from the Sun.
PLUTO	The ninth planet from the Sun. The God of the Underworld in the classical myths.
RETROGRADE	A term describing periods when a planet appears to move backwards in the sky.
QUADRUPLICITY	A division of the Zodiac into groups of four signs corresponding to the Qualities, Cardinal, Fixed and Mutable (q.v.).
QUALITY	One of the three characteristics shown by a sign (see CARDINAL, FIXED and MUTABLE).

SAGITTARIUS	The Archer. The ninth sign of the Zodiac.
SATURN	The sixth planet from the Sun and the last that can be observed by the unaided eye. The keeper of time, structure and boundaries in classical mythology.
SCORPIO	The Scorpion. The eighth sign of the Zodiac.
SEXTILE	An Aspect where two planets are 60^0 apart, seen as harmonious, often with a practical outcome.
SIGN	One of the signs of the Zodiac, named after 12 constellations lying along an imaginary belt around the Earth. (See ARIES, TAURUS, GEMINI, CANCER, LEO, VIRGO, LIBRA, SCORPIO, SAGITTARIUS, CAPRICORN, AQUARIUS and PISCES.)
SQUARE	An Aspect in which two planets are at 90^0 to each other. Generally regarded as a 'hard' aspect, it draws attention to issues that need to be dealt with.
TAURUS	The Bull. The second sign of the Zodiac.
TRANSIT	The relationship between a planet's actual position in the sky at a specific moment, and the position of itself or any other planet at the time of birth. Transits often mark important life events.

TRINE
An Aspect in which two planets, or a planet and an Angle are 120° apart. A 'soft' aspect, indicating an easy flow of energies between the planets involved.

TRIPLICITY
A division of the Zodiac into groups of three signs, each characterised by one of the Elements (q.v.).

URANUS
The seventh planet from the Sun, and the first to be discovered by observation with a telescope.
In mythology, a Titan and father of Saturn.

VENUS
The second planet from the Sun.
The Goddess of Love, beauty and the arts in classical mythology.

VIRGO
The Young Woman. The sixth sign of the Zodiac.

ZODIAC
An imaginary belt around the Earth on which the 12 signs are located.

★ BIBLIOGRAPHY

Gods and Planets	Ellynor Barz, Chiron Publications, 1993
A Woman's Herbal	Elisabeth Brooke, The Women's Press, 1992
The New Astrology	Nicolas Campion & Steve Eddy, Bloomsbury, 1999
Chiron	Barbara Hand Clow, Llewellyn Publications, 1993
The Astrological Judgement of Diseases	Nicholas Culpeper, Ascella Publications, 1655
The Herbal	Nicholas Culpeper, Wordsworth Editions Ltd, 1995
Magical Aromatherapy	Scott Cunningham, Llewellyn Publications, 1989
Asteroid Goddesses	Demetra George, ACS Publications, 1986
Planetary Aspects	Tracey Marks, CRCS Publications, 1987
The Art of Timing	J. Paungger & T. Poppe, The C.W. Daniel Co. Ltd, 2000
The Gods of Change	Howard Sasportas, Arkana, 1989
The Twelve Houses	Howard Sasportas, The Aquarian Press, 1985
Culpeper's Medicine	Graeme Tobyn, Element, 1997
Plantes Medicinales	J. Volak & J. Stodola, eds. Grund, Paris, 1983
The Art of Aromatherapy	Robert Tisserand, The C.W. Daniel Co. Ltd, 1977
Herbs in Magic and Alchemy	C.L. Zalewski, Prisms Press, 1999

★ RECOMMENDED FURTHER READING

BOOKS ABOUT AROMATHERAPY – INTRODUCTORY

Aromatherapy during your Pregnancy	Frances R. Clifford, The C.W. Daniel Co. Ltd, 1997
Aromatherapy, An A-Z	Patricia Davis, The C.W. Daniel Co. Ltd, 1988
First Steps in Aromatherapy	Jane Dye, The C.W. Daniel Co. Ltd, 1996
Aromatherapy for Women and Children	Jane Dye, The C.W. Daniel Co. Ltd, 1992
The Encyclopedia of Essential Oils	Julia Lawless, Element Books Ltd, 1992

BOOKS ABOUT AROMATHERAPY – CONTINUATION

Subtle Aromatherapy	Patricia Davis, The C.W. Daniel Co. Ltd, 1991
Gattefossés Aromatherapy	R.M. Gattefossé, The C.W. Daniel Co. Ltd, 1993
Marguerite Maury's Guide to Aromatherapy	Marguerite Maury, The C.W. Daniel Co. Ltd, 1989
Aromatherapy for Healing the Spirit	Gabriel Mojay, Gaia Books Ltd, 1996
The Practice of Aromatherapy	Jean Valnet, The C.W. Daniel Co. Ltd, 1980

BOOKS ABOUT ASTROLOGY – INTRODUCTORY

A Journey Round the Birthchart	Joanne Wickenburg, CRCS Publications, 1985
The Round Art	A.T. Mann, Dragon's World Ltd, 1979
The New Astrology	Nicolas Campion & Steve Eddy, Bloomsbury, 1999

BOOKS ABOUT ASTROLOGY - CONTINUATION

Gods and Planets	Ellynor Barz, Chiron Publications, 1993
Chiron	Barbara Hand Clow, Llewellyn Publications, 1993
Asteroid Goddesses	Demetra George, ACS Publications, 1986
The Gods of Change	Howard Sasportas, Arkana, 1989
The Twelve Houses	Howard Sasportas, The Aquarian Press, 1985
The Consultation Chart	Wanda Sellar, Wessex Astrologer, 2001

BOOKS ABOUT MEDICAL ASTROLOGY

The Astrological Judgement of Diseases	Nicholas Culpeper, Ascella Publications, 1655
A Handbook of Medical Astrology	Jane Ridder-Patrick, Arkana, 1990

AROMATHERAPY TRAINING UK and overseas

THE INTERNATIONAL FEDERATION OF PROFESSIONAL AROMATHERAPISTS,

182 Chiswick High Road,

LONDON

W4 1PP

National body for aromatherapy in the UK, amalgamating the former International Federation of Aromatherapists, International Society of Professional Aromatherapists and the Register of Qualified Aromatherapists. Send s.a.e. for list of accredited courses in UK and overseas, also for details of qualified aromatherapists in your locality.

LONDON SCHOOL OF AROMATHERAPY (L.S.A. NORTH)

PO Box 11850,

Turriff,

ABERDEEN,

AB53 8YA

Freephone: 0800 716 847

Aromatherapy courses designed by the author. Send s.a.e. for details of training in London, other areas of the UK and overseas.

FRAGRANT STUDIES,

The Pilgrims Centre,

Orchard Court,

Magdalene Street,

GLASTONBURY,

BA6 9EW

Tel: 01458 835920

email: fragrant-studies@fragrant-earth.com

Courses and seminars in Glastonbury, Scotland and elsewhere.

AROMATHERAPY TRAINING USA

FINGER LAKES SCHOOL OF MASSAGE,

1251 Trumansburg Road,

Ithaca NY, 14850

USA

Tel: 607-272-9024

email: admissions@flsm.com

INSTITUTE OF AROMATHERAPY,

3108 Route 10 West,

DENVILLE,

NJ 07834,

USA

Tel: 973-989-1999

email: essence@aromatherapy4u.com

NATIONAL ASSOCIATION OF HOLISTIC AROMATHERAPISTS, (NAHA)

4509 Interlake Avenue N., 233,

SEATTLE,

WA 98103-6773,

USA

Tel: 206-547-2164

email: info@NAHA.org

Holds details of courses and practitioners.

ESSENTIAL OIL SUPPLIERS IRELAND & UK

ABSOLUTE ESSENTIALS,

Derrynaneal,

FEAKLE,

Co. Clare,

Ireland

email: absolute@esatclear.ie

Organic and wild-grown essential oils. Mail-order to UK and most countries.

AQUA OLEUM,
Unit 3,
Lower Wharf,
Wallbridge,
STROUD,
GL5 3JA
Tel: 01453 753555
A range of organic oils by mail order and in some health-food shops. Also non-organic but good quality oils widely available in health-food stores.

FRAGRANT EARTH,
Orchard Court,
Magdalene Street,
GLASTONBURY,
BA6 9EW
Tel: 01458 831216
email: all-enquiries@fragrant-earth.com
Very wide range of organic and wild-grown oils, carrier oils, bases, etc. Mail order only.

ESSENTIAL OIL SUPPLIERS USA

AROMATHERAPY INSTITUTE & RESEARCH,
PO Box 2354,
FAIR OAKS,
CA 95628,
USA
Tel: 916-965-7546
email: leydet@leydet.com

ASTROLOGICAL ORGANISATIONS UK

THE ASTROLOGICAL ASSOCIATION,
Unit 168,
Lee Valley Technopark,
Tottenham Hale,
LONDON
N17 5TN
Tel: 020 8880 4848
email: astrological.association@zetnet.co.uk
Organises seminars, workshops and an annual conference. Publishes bi-monthly journal and several bi-annual specialist journals. Also publishes Astrology and Medicine Newsletter from a separate address (see below). Open to all - professional astrologers and lay members.

ASTROLOGY AND MEDICINE NEWSLETTER,
8 Swan Grove,
Chappel,
Essex,
CO6 2DU
Thrice-yearly newsletter of special interest to people working with astrology and healing.

ASTROLOGICAL LODGE OF LONDON,
50 Gloucester Place,
LONDON
W1H 4EA
Offers regular programme of lectures and classes (beginners' classes are free of charge) and publishes quarterly journal.

FACULTY OF ASTROLOGICAL STUDIES,
BM Box 7470,
LONDON
WC1N 3XX
Tel: 07000 790143
email: info@astrology.org.uk
Day and evening classes in London plus distance learning courses at all levels. Weekend seminars and annual summer school. Online tuition planned in near future. Publishes student newsletter.

THE LONDON SCHOOL OF ASTROLOGY,
BCM Planets,
LONDON
WC1N 3XX
Tel: 00700 233 44 55
email: admin@londonschoolofastrology.co.uk
website: www.londonschoolofastrology.co.uk
Classes at foundation and advanced levels, seminars, lectures and summer schools. Emphasis on the holistic and spiritual aspects of astrology.

URANIA TRUST,
12 Warrington Spur,
OLD WINDSOR,
Berks
SL4 2NF
Tel: 01753 851107
email: urania.trust@ntlworld.com
Encourages the study of all branches of astrology. Fosters links with related fields, and astrologers in other countries. Publishes specialised books, etc.

ASTROLOGICAL ORGANISATIONS OVERSEAS

Australia

AUSTRALIAN SOCIETY OF ASTROLOGERS,
PO Box 7120,
Bass Hill,
New South Wales, 2197,
Australia
email: GJdeMAS@bigpond.com.au
Encourages flexibility and individual development of members. Publishes bi-monthly newsletter.

FEDERATION OF AUSTRALIAN ASTROLOGERS,
National Secretary: Sylvia Wilson,
PO Box 466,
Wood Ridge,
Queensland,
Australia
email: Sylvia@powerup.com.au
Has branches in each of the states. Publishes professional journal.

Canada

CANADIAN ACADEMY OF ASTROLOGY AND RELATED DISCIPLINES,
Tel: (613) 722-5975
email: cyclespeak@aol.com
(No other information available)

Ireland

THE ASTROLOGICAL FEDERATION OF IRELAND,
Secretary: Rink Condrat,
New Haggard,
Lusk, Co. Dublin,
Ireland
Organises regular lectures, workshops, etc.

THE IRISH ASTROLOGICAL ASSOCIATION,

Contact: Kay Doyle,

193 Lower Rathmines Road,

Rathmines,

Dublin 6,

Ireland

Organises weekly classes and lectures and annual conference.

New Zealand

ASTROLOGICAL SOCIETY OF NEW ZEALAND,

PO Box 5266,

Wellesley Street,

AUCKLAND C1,

New Zealand

Tel: 064 09 480-8019

email: clearvu@ihug.co.nz

Organises conferences, publishes quarterly magazine, has library of books and tape and aims to facilitate contact between astrologers in New Zealand and abroad.

South Africa

ASTROLOGICAL SOCIETY OF SOUTH AFRICA,

Contact: Elena van Baalen

PO Box 1953,

Saxonwold 2132

South Africa

email: elena@kallback.co.za

USA

AMERICAN FEDERATION OF ASTROLOGERS,

PO Box 22040,

Tempe,

AZ 85285-2040,

USA

email: afa@msn.com

Organises conventions, workshops and examinations, holds extensive library of data and astrological books.

ASTROLOGICAL INSTITUTE,

7501 E. Oak Street,

Suite 130,

SCOTTSDALE,

AZ 85257,

USA

Tel: 480 423-9494

email: astroin@primenet.com

State accredited courses in astrology and psychology.

THE INTERNATIONAL SOCIETY OF ASTROLOGICAL RESEARCH,

PO Box 38613,

LOS ANGELES,

CA 90038-0613,

USA

email: maribiehn@hotmail.com

Promotes astrological research, publishes books and quarterly journal, organises seminars and conferences.

ASTROLOGY SOFTWARE SUPPLIERS UK

MATRIX SOFTWARE,
Old Post Office House,
Main Street,
Tyninghame,
DUNBAR,
EH42 1XL
Tel: 01620 861717
email: martin@matrixastrology.com

ROY GILLETT CONSULTANTS,
32 Glynswood,
CAMBERLEY,
Surrey
GU15 1HU
Tel: 01276 683898
email: roy.gillett@dial.pipex.com

ASTROLOGY SOFTWARE SUPPLIERS USA

MICROCYCLES,
PO Box 3175
CULVER CITY,
CA 90231,
USA
Tel: 1-800-829-2537
website: www.microcycles.com

MATRIX SOFTWARE,
4407 N. State Street,
BIG RAPIDS,
MI 49307,
USA
Tel: 231-796-6343
website: http://www.astrologysoftware.com

TIME CYCLES RESEARCH,
375 Willetts Avenue,
WATERFORD,
CT 06385,
USA
Tel: 800-827-2240
email: astrology@timecycles.com

★ INDEX